Handbook for Prescribing Medications During Pregnancy

Handbook for Prescribing Medications During Pregnancy

Edited by

Richard L. Berkowitz, M.D., M.P.H.

Associate Professor of Obstetrics
and Gynecology and of Public Health,
Yale University School of Medicine;
Director, High Risk Obstetrical Service,
Yale–New Haven Medical Center,
New Haven

Donald R. Coustan, M.D.

Associate Professor of Obstetrics and Gynecology,
Yale University School of Medicine;
Attending Perinatologist,
High Risk Obstetrical Service,
Yale–New Haven Medical Center,
New Haven

Tara K. Mochizuki, Pharm.D.

Assistant Clinical Professor of Pharmacy,
University of California, San Francisco,
School of Medicine;
Staff Pharmacist,
University of California Medical Center,
San Diego

Little, Brown and Company • Boston

Library of Congress Catalog Card No. 80-83310

ISBN 0-316-09173-1

Printed in the United States of America

HAL

To **Nathan G. Kase, M.D. and John C. Hobbins, M.D.,**
Our Mentors, Colleagues, and Friends

Contents

Preface

This book was inspired by the frequent phone calls received by each of the editors regarding the administering of drugs to pregnant women. Its purpose is to provide clinicians with an up-to-date desktop reference on the use of drugs during pregnancy. The publication of new data in multiple journals makes it very difficult to stay abreast of current work in this dynamic field. Furthermore, no major reference work has been devoted specifically to this subject. Since the pharmacological actions of drugs administered during pregnancy may have effects that reach far beyond the therapeutic intent for which they were prescribed, few areas of information have more practical importance.

Because of the bewildering variety of pharmacological preparations currently available in the United States, we have made no attempt to be comprehensive. Instead we have tried to select widely available and frequently prescribed preparations as well as those specifically indicated for uncommon conditions that can affect obstetrical patients. We have also included discussions of some drugs that are not indicated during pregnancy because they might be inadvertently taken before conception has been confirmed.

This book is not intended to rival standard pharmacological textbooks in terms of detailed descriptions of mechanisms of action, metabolic degradation pathways, stoichiometric parameters, and the like. It is a synopsis of the most current relevant information about the effects of individual drugs on the pregnant woman. In addition, we have attempted to present data concerning both the mutagenic and teratogenic potential of each agent on the developing fetus. Each entry begins with the indications for use of that particular drug and the author's specific recommendations. If the drug is absolutely contraindicated during pregnancy, or relatively contraindicated because other therapeutic agents are preferable, this is stated and explained. Drugs that do not fall into these categories are divided into those that are (1) safe for use during pregnancy, (2) indicated only for specific conditions, or (3) the subject of ongoing controversy. In any of these cases a further discussion ensues. A section on special considerations during pregnancy discusses effects that are specifically related to the pregnancy. These include sequelae to both mother and fetus as well as the impact on breastfeeding infants. Appropriate dosages are then presented, followed by a listing of potential general adverse effects. The drug's pharmacological properties are next described in terms of major mechanisms of action, and its absorption and biotransformation are summarized. Finally, each entry concludes with a few relevant recommended readings.

The problems of studying the effects on the fetus of drugs administered to the mother are formidable. In many cases this information is simply not known. Many pharmacological agents have been released by the FDA without specific approval for use during pregnancy. The *Physicians' Desk Reference* frequently offers the familiar caveat: "The safety of _____ in human pregnancy has not been established. The use of the drug in pregnancy requires that the expected therapeutic benefit be weighed against possible hazard to mother and infant." This is not terribly helpful. Obviously, pharmacological agents should not be given during the first trimester, when embryogenesis is occurring, unless absolutely necessary. Another important principle, however, is that medically indicated drug therapy should not be withheld from pregnant women. We have offered specific recommendations about the advisability of utilizing particular drugs with the understanding that they never should be administered frivolously during pregnancy. Our suggestions are based on currently available information, and they may need revision as more is learned. Furthermore, despite our efforts to be thorough, it is certainly possible that some published reports may have escaped our attention. We plan to continue to maintain an active surveillance of the literature and hope to update the material with subsequent editions. If a reader is aware of any data that have been overlooked, he or she should not hesitate to contact the editors so that appropriate additions can be made in the future.

Our approach has been to consider each drug individually. We have not tried to write a manual of therapeutics. Consequently, this book is not particularly intended for the reader who is attempting to formulate a treatment plan for a specific complex problem, such as asthma or hypertension. If, however, the reader is interested in knowing whether a particular drug, such as ephedrine, should be prescribed for the pregnant asthmatic, this can quickly be determined. If a drug is not recommended because another one is considered preferable, the preferred alternative is cited.

The entries are arranged alphabetically by generic name. Some of the more common brand names are also presented with each drug. A general index includes both generic and trade names, while a classification index subdivides the drugs into functional groups by generic name only. Groups of related drugs, such as the penicillins, are sometimes presented in a single entry. The individual constituents of these families, however, are listed separately in the general index and are also considered independently within the entry when this is warranted. Over-the-counter (OTC) preparations are listed according to their major generic ingredients. Tobacco, alcohol (ethyl), and marijuana are separate entries. Vitamin and mineral requirements during pregnancy are discussed in the Appendix.

The individual entries were prepared by house staff and faculty members in the Department of Obstetrics and Gynecology of the Yale University School of Medicine and staff members of the Department of Pharmacy Services of the Yale–New Haven Medical Center. (The author's initials can be found in parentheses following each entry.) All entries were reviewed by the three editors, two of whom are practicing perinatologists, while the third is a clinical pharmacist. Some recommendations concerning drug preference, dosage schedules, and routes of administration reflect appraoches that are utilized on the obstetric service of the Yale–New Haven Medical Center, in preference to other acceptable alternatives. Whenever this is the case, it has been so stated in the text.

R.L.B.
D.R.C.
T.K.M.

Contributors

Richard L. Berkowitz, M.D. *(RLB)*
Elizabeth A. Capriotti, R.Ph. *(EAC)*
John R. Cote, Pharm.D. *(JRC)*
Donald R. Coustan, M.D. *(DRC)*
Ronald A. Cwik, M.D. *(RAC)*
Alan H. DeCherney, M.D. *(AHD)*
Greggory R. DeVore, M.D. *(GRD)*
Allan D. DiCamillo, R.Ph. *(ADD)*
Arnold J. Friedman, M.D. *(AJF)*
Joel A. Giuditta, R.Ph. *(JAG)*
Peter A. Grannum, M.D. *(PAG)*
Robert J. Harrison, R.Ph. *(RJH)*
Thomas K. Hazlet, Pharm.D. *(TKH)*
Joyce M. Heineman, R.Ph. *(JMH)*
Brian D. Hotchkiss, R.Ph. *(BDH)*
David J. Iamkis, R.Ph. *(DJI)*
Daniel J. Kazienko, R.Ph. *(DJK)*
Phyllis C. Leppert, M.D. *(PCL)*
Mark C. Malzer, M.D. *(MCM)*
Mary Jane Minkin, M.D. *(MJM)*
Tara K. Mochizuki, Pharm.D. *(TKM)*
William O'Brien, M.D. *(WO'B)*
Phillip H. Radell, M.D. *(PHR)*
Peter L. Ricupero. R.Ph. *(PLR)*
Roberto J. Romero, M.D. *(RJR)*
Paul J. Roszko, R.Ph. *(PJR)*
Bonnie R. Saks, M.D. *(BRS)*
C. Robert Sturwold, R.Ph. *(CRS)*
Khalil Tabsh, M.D. *(KT)*
C. Edward Todd, R.Ph. *(CET)*
Ellen M. Todesca, R.Ph. *(EMT)*
Cecily R. Victor, R.Ph. *(CRV)*

Notice

Acetaminophen (Datril®, Nebs®, Tempra®, Tylenol®)

INDICATIONS AND RECOMMENDATIONS

Acetaminophen is safe to use during pregnancy in therapeutic dosages. Although this compound does cross the placenta, available evidence suggests that congenital malformations are not associated with maternal use. The use of large doses by pregnant women, however, can result in fetal renal changes similar to those seen in adults. Maternal overusage may cause significant sequelae, including hepatic necrosis. Because of concern about the antiplatelet activity of aspirin, however, acetaminophen is the analgesic and antipyretic of choice during pregnancy.

SPECIAL CONSIDERATIONS IN PREGNANCY

There are no unique maternal problems when acetaminophen is taken during pregnancy. Although it crosses the placenta, no adverse effects on the fetus have been reported. Fetal hemolytic anemia and methemoglobinemia are theoretical possibilities but are very unlikely since a single 2-gram dose converts less than 3% of the total circulating hemoglobin to methemoglobin, a level of methemoglobin of little clinical significance. Renal abnormalities were noted in a newborn whose mother ingested 1.3 gm of acetaminophen daily throughout the pregnancy.

DOSAGE

The usual dose of acetaminophen is 325–650 mg every 4 hours, with a maximum dose of 2.6 gm/day. The drug comes in tablets (120, 325, and 650 mg), and in elixir and syrup (120 mg/5 ml).

ADVERSE EFFECTS

A variety of central nervous system (CNS) symptoms have been attributed to acetaminophen, including relaxation and drowsiness as well as stimulation and euphoria. Patients occasionally complain of lightheadedness, dizziness, and a sense of unreality and detachment. An erythematous or urticarial skin rash associated with a drug fever can occur. Idiosyncratic responses include neutropenia, leukopenia, pancytopenia, and thrombocytopenia. Methemoglobinemia and hemolytic anemia may occur as acute toxic reactions, but they are usually seen in association with chronic overdosage. Hepatic necrosis may also occur with overdosage. Nephrotoxicity secondary to papillary necrosis and chronic interstitial nephritis have been described in chronic abusers. Excessive ingestion can also cause hypoglycemic coma and myocardial damage.

MECHANISM OF ACTION

Both the antipyretic and analgesic actions of this drug seem to be due to a direct hypothalamic effect. The effect of endogenous pyrogens on CNS heat regulatory centers is inhibited, and this results in peripheral vasodilation with subsequent loss of body heat. The analgesic actions are less well understood.

ABSORPTION AND BIOTRANSFORMATION

Acetaminophen becomes evenly distributed among all body fluids. Approximately 3% is excreted unchanged in the urine while 80% is conjugated with glucuronic acid and then excreted by the kidneys. Hydroxylated metabolites form a conjugate, and it is this complex that is responsible for methemoglobin formation, hepatic toxicity, and red blood cell hemolysis.

This drug is rapidly absorbed from the gastrointestinal tract and reaches peak plasma concentration in ½–1 hour. The plasma half-life is 1–3 hours.

RECOMMENDED READING

Goodman, L. S., and Gilman, A.   *The Pharmacological Basis of Therapeutics* (5th ed.). New York: Macmillan, 1975. Pp. 343–348.

Nelson, M. M., and Forfar, J. O.   Associations between drugs administered during pregnancy and congenital abnormalities of the fetus. *Br. Med. J.* 1:523–527, 1971.

Schenkel, B., and Vorherr, H.   Non-prescription drugs during pregnancy: Potential teratogenic and toxic effects upon embryo and fetus. *J. Reprod. Med.* 12:27–45, 1974.

(RAC)

Acetazolamide (Diamox®)

INDICATIONS AND RECOMMENDATIONS

The use of acetazolamide during pregnancy should be limited to adjunctive therapy for increased intraocular pressure and the treatment of increased intracranial pressure caused by pseudotumor cerebri. It may also be used in the prophylactic management of petit mal epilepsy in women whose seizures increase at the time of menstruation. Although animal data implicate the drug as a teratogen, no human data support this. Periodic monitoring of electrolyte balance is recommended when this drug is given during pregnancy.

SPECIAL CONSIDERATIONS IN PREGNANCY

Acetazolamide has been shown to cause forelimb malformations in some offspring of pregnant rats receiving doses of 200 mg/kg. This is greater than ten times the usual adult human dose. As of yet, retrospective data have not shown any significant incidence of malformations in infants whose mothers have received therapeutic doses of acetazolamide during pregnancy. It is not known whether acetazolamide enters human breast milk.

DOSAGE

The recommended adult dose of acetazolamide for adjunctive treatment of open-angle glaucoma is 250 mg taken orally qd to qid or a 500 mg sustained-release capsule taken bid. For rapid lowering of intraocular pressure, 500 mg may be given parenterally. As an adjunct in the prophylactic management of epilepsy, the usual oral dosage is 250 mg qd in addition to other anticonvulsants.

ADVERSE EFFECTS

Serious side effects are rare. Most adverse reactions are dose-dependent and usually respond to a decrease in the amount being administered or to withdrawal of the drug. Patients may experience drowsiness, temporary myopia, skin rashes, anorexia, and nausea. The most common side effects are changes in fluid and electrolyte balance, especially metabolic acidosis and hypokalemia. More serious, but rarer, adverse reactions include hypersensitivity reactions, bone marrow depression, and renal toxicity.

MECHANISM OF ACTION

Acetazolamide acts by a noncompetitive inhibition of carbonic anhydrase to reduce the formation of hydrogen ion and bicarbonate ion from carbon dioxide and water. This inhibition results in decreased production of aqueous humor, increased renal excretion of bicarbonate ion with alkalinization of the urine, and increased excretion of sodium and potassium with resultant diuresis. Plasma bicarbonate is decreased and plasma chloride increased.

The anticonvulsant activity of acetazolamide is thought to be due to the induced metabolic acidosis. Another postulated mechanism is a direct action on the brain by increased carbon dioxide tension, which has been shown to retard neuronal conduction. In addition, cerebrospinal fluid formation may be decreased.

ABSORPTION AND BIOTRANSFORMATION

Acetazolamide is readily absorbed from the gastrointestinal tract with peak plasma concentrations occurring within 2 hours. Onset of action after an oral dose is approximately 1 hour later, while its duration is 8–12 hours. A time-release preparation is available, the duration of which is 18–24 hours. When given intravenously, onset of action occurs within 2 minutes, peak effect occurs at 15 minutes, and duration is 4–5 hours. Its major route of elimination is via the kidney where it undergoes active tubular secretion.

RECOMMENDED READING

Goodman, L. S., and Gilman, A. *The Pharmacological Basis of Therapeutics* (5th ed.). New York: Macmillan, 1975. Pp. 218–221.

Heinonen, O. P., Slone, D., and Shapiro, S. *Birth Defects and Drugs in Pregnancy*. Littleton, Mass.: Publishing Sciences Group, 1977. Pp. 372, 441, 495.

Layton, W., and Hallesy, D. W. Deformity of forelimb in rats: Association with high doses of acetazolamide. *Science* 149:306–308, 1965.

Long, J. W. *The Essential Guide to Prescription Drugs*. New York: Harper & Row, 1977. Pp. 265–267.

(DJK)

Albumin (Albuminar®, Albuspan®, Albutein®)

INDICATIONS AND RECOMMENDATIONS

The use of albumin during pregnancy should be limited to the treatment of acute oliguria secondary to hypovolemia. It can also be used as a temporary plasma expander during hypovolemic states secondary to hemorrhage if blood is not immediately available. Central venous pressure should be carefully monitored when albumin is administered during pregnancy.

SPECIAL CONSIDERATIONS IN PREGNANCY

Albumin does not cross the placenta. Pregnancy is generally accompanied by an increase in maternal intravascular volume; in severe pregnancy-induced hypertension, however, hypovolemia often occurs. In this situation, albumin may occasionally be used to increase oncotic pressure and improve renal perfusion. If albumin is given, central pressures should be monitored in order to document hypovolemia and to prevent the development of heart failure due to secondary intravascular overload.

DOSAGE

Albumin is supplied in 25% solution, with 50 ml containing 12.5 gm of albumin and 100 ml containing 25 gm. The onset of action is immediate since it is given intravenously.

ADVERSE EFFECTS

Albumin is inert. The major side effect is intravascular overload, especially in the patient with compromised cardiovascular status; congestive heart failure may occur in this setting.

MECHANISM OF ACTION

Normal human serum albumin is a sterile preparation from the fractionated blood of healthy donors. It is generally free of the hepatitis virus.

The intravenous administration of albumin raises the oncotic pressure of the intravascular space. Extracellular fluid is thus drawn into the intravascular compartment. Hypotension is improved, and renal perfusion is increased, with a resultant increase in urinary output.

RECOMMENDED READING

Gifford, R. W., Jr. A guide to the practical use of diuretics. *J.A.M.A.* 235:1890–1893, 1976.

Goodman, L. S., and Gilman, A. *The Pharmacological Basis of Therapeutics* (5th ed.). New York: Macmillan, 1975. P. 769.

Pritchard, J., and MacDonald, P. *Williams Obstetrics* (15th ed.). New York: Appleton-Century-Crofts, 1976. Pp. 551–581.

(PCL)

Alcohol, Ethyl (Ethanol)

INDICATIONS AND RECOMMENDATIONS

Ethyl alcohol may be administered to pregnant women for the treatment of premature labor. It is also taken socially, but its chronic use has been associated with a constellation of fetal anomalies. Although chronic alcohol ingestion is absolutely contraindicated throughout pregnancy, there are not enough data available to determine whether the occasional social drink is harmful to the fetus. No recommendation can therefore be made in regard to social drinking during pregnancy. Although ethanol may be effective in the treatment of premature labor in the third trimester, beta mimetic agents are probably a better choice in this situation.

SPECIAL CONSIDERATIONS IN PREGNANCY

Chronic ethanol ingestion has been associated with the fetal alcohol syndrome, which consists of prenatal-onset growth deficiency, developmental delay, craniofacial anomalies, incomplete development of cerebral cortex, microcephaly, and maxillary hypoplasia. It is not yet clear whether alcohol itself, or its metabolite acetaldehyde, is acting as the toxin to produce abnormalities. Both substances cross the placenta, and in animal studies both affect somites, deforming the brain and spinal cord and producing severe growth retardation. The quantity and regularity of alcohol consumption around conception and during various stages of pregnancy in women may have different effects. It is likely that heavy drinking during the first trimester has the greatest effect on fetal maldevelopment, whereas excessive alcohol consumption later in the pregnancy may have greater effect on fetal nutrition and size.

Recent studies indicate that chronic alcohol ingestion of greater than 2.2 gm of absolute alcohol/kg/day increases the frequency of all abnormalities associated with the fetal alcohol syndrome. This quantity is the approximate equivalent of 4½ ounces of pure alcohol, or 9 ounces of 100 proof liquor, or 1¼ liters of 12% table wine daily.

Ethanol has been used in the treatment of premature labor in the third trimester, although beta mimetic agents are probably a better choice in this situation. Because alcohol is still used in many centers for this purpose, a protocol for stopping premature labor will be included in this section.

DOSAGE

Before alcohol infusion is begun, the patient should be thoroughly checked for conditions such as premature rupture of membranes, abruptio placentae, or urinary tract infection, any one of which may be causative of the premature labor. In the treatment of uncomplicated premature labor an intravenous loading dose of 7.5 mg/kg/hour is given over 2 hours, followed by a maintenance dose of 1.5

mg/kg/hour given over 10 hours. Premature labor usually responds to a single course of intravenous alcohol. The onset and duration of action varies in each individual patient. Alcohol will be present in the bloodstream for 10–12 hours after the infusion is stopped.

ADVERSE EFFECTS

Side effects of alcohol consumption include nausea and vomiting (with the potential for aspiration pneumonia), hypoglycemia, central nervous system depression, and mild hypotension. These effects are seen whether the alcohol is taken orally or intravenously (as in the treatment of premature labor). The complications of excessive consumption include increased blood lactate, hyperlipemia, and fatty liver. The continued use of large amounts of alcohol can lead to alcoholic hepatitis and cirrhosis. There are, however, individual differences in response to alcohol; in particular, not all heavy drinkers develop hepatitis and cirrhosis.

MECHANISM OF ACTION

Ethanol inhibits release of the neurohypophyseal hormones oxytocin and vasopressin from the posterior pituitary gland. Intravenous or oral administration in early premature labor (with intact membranes) will postpone labor in two-thirds of cases. This is somewhat better than results in women in control groups who were given intravenous glucose. It is assumed that the effect of alcohol on labor is due to inhibition of oxytocin release.

The central nervous system is most markedly affected with the social ingestion of alcohol. Ethanol is a primary and continuous depressant of the central nervous system. The apparent stimulation gained from social drinking results from the unrestrained activity of parts of the brain when inhibitory control mechanisms for those parts are depressed. It is this "stimulation" that gives ethanol-containing products their high potential for abuse. Other physiological effects include vasodilation, stimulation of gastric secretions, and diuresis due to inhibition of the antidiuretic hormone.

ABSORPTION AND BIOTRANSFORMATION

Ethyl alcohol is absorbed from the stomach, small intestine, and colon. Absorption from the small intestine is rapid and complete. In the liver, ethanol is metabolized to acetaldehyde at a rate of 10 ml/hour. Acetaldehyde is then normally oxidized to acetyl coenzyme A, which is in turn metabolized in the citric acid cycle.

RECOMMENDED READING

Hanson, J. W., Jones, K. L., and Smith, D. W. Fetal alcohol syndrome. *J.A.M.A.* 235:1458–1460, 1976.

Jones, K. L., and Smith, D. W. The fetal alcoholic syndrome. *Teratology* 12:1–10, 1975.

Jones, K. L., Smith, D. W., Streissouth, A. P., and Myrianthopoulos, N. C. Outcome in offspring of chronic alcoholic women. *Lancet* 1:95–96, 1974.

Lieber, C. S. Metabolism of alcohol. *Sci. Am.* 234:25–33, 1976.

Ouellette, E., Rosetti, H. L., Rosman, N. P., and Weiner, L. Adverse effects on offspring of maternal alcohol abuse during pregnancy. *N. Engl. J. Med.* 297:528–530, 1977.

Palmer, R. H., Ouellette, E. M., Warner, L., and Leichtman, S. R. Congenital malformations in offspring of a chronic alcoholic mother. *Pediatrics* 53:490–494, 1974.

(PAG)

Allopurinol (Zyloprim®)

INDICATIONS AND RECOMMENDATIONS

The use of allopurinol is relatively contraindicated during pregnancy because other therapeutic agents are preferable (for example, probenecid). It is used for the treatment of both the primary hyperuricemia of gout and hyperuricemia secondary to hematological disorders and antineoplastic therapy.

Allopurinol and its metabolite, alloxanthine, inhibit xanthine oxidase, the enzyme that catalyzes the conversion of hypoxanthine to xanthine and xanthine to uric acid. Thus, serum and urine levels of uric acid are decreased while levels of the more soluble oxypurine precursors are increased. The decrease in serum urate levels occurs during the first 1 to 3 weeks of therapy.

Attacks of gout may occur more frequently during the initial months of therapy. Hypersensitivity reactions, predominantly erythematous, pruritic, or maculopapular cutaneous eruptions may occur. Occasionally these lesions may be exfoliative, urticarial, or purpuric. Fever, malaise, and muscle aches may also become manifest. Transient leukopenia, leukocytosis, or eosinophilia are rare reactions but may require cessation of therapy. Headache, drowsiness, nausea and vomiting, diarrhea, and gastric irritation occur occasionally.

Allopurinol is not teratogenic in mice. Due to its structural similarity to purines, there is a theoretical possibility that this drug or one of its metabolites may be incorporated into nucleic acids. It has been shown, however, that neither allopurinol nor alloxanthine are incorporated into DNA during any stage of replication and that they produce no mutagenic effect. Allopurinol's effects on the human fetus are unknown.

Gout is uncommon in women and is rarely seen before menopause. Elevated serum uric acid is common in toxemia but rarely requires therapy. Probenecid has been safely used and is indicated for treatment of hyperuricemia in pregnancy.

RECOMMENDED READING

Burrow, G. N., and Ferris, T. F. (Eds.). *Medical Complications During Pregnancy.* New York: Saunders, 1975. P. 805.

Goodman, L. S., and Gilman, A. *The Pharmacological Basis of Therapeutics* (5th ed.). New York: Macmillan, 1975. Pp. 352–354.

Stevenson, A. C., Silcock, S. R., and Scott, J. T. Absence of chromosome damage in human lymphocytes exposed to allopurinol and oxipurinol. *Ann. Rheum. Dis.* 35:143–147, 1976.

(CRV)

Alphaprodine (Nisentil®)

INDICATIONS AND RECOMMENDATIONS

Alphaprodine may be used as an analgesic in patients in the active phase of labor at term. A synthetic narcotic indicated for the relief of moderate to severe pain, its onset of action is faster than that of morphine or meperidine when given subcutaneously but its duration of analgesia is shorter. In most cases there is no significant advantage to using alphaprodine rather than morphine or meperidine. The safe use of alphaprodine in pregnancy, other than during labor, has not been established.

It is recommended that if this drug is used during labor, the lowest effective dose should be administered. Infants born to mothers who have received alphaprodine as antepartum analgesia should be observed for respiratory depression. Should this occur it can be reversed by naloxone.

The degree of neonatal respiratory depression produced by any narcotic administered during labor depends on the gestational age and condition of the infant. The magnitude of this effect is inversely proportional to gestational age and may be potentiated by birth asphyxia. Alphaprodine, therefore, should be used with extreme caution, if at all, during a labor that will produce a premature infant.

SPECIAL CONSIDERATIONS IN PREGNANCY

Most clinical reports indicate that alphaprodine does not interfere with the active phase of labor. *Any* narcotic administered during the latent phase, however, may result in uterine inertia. When meperidine was compared to alphaprodine in one study no significant difference in duration of labor was noted.

All narcotics cross the placental barrier, and neonatal respiratory depression has been seen with the use of alphaprodine during labor. This may be due to vasoconstriction of placental vessels, as well as to a direct depressant effect on the infant's respiratory center. Bonica states that the degree of neonatal depression caused by all narcotics during their peak action is about the same when the drug is given to the mother in equianalgesic doses. The peak effect of most narcotics following subcutaneous or intramuscular administration is seen in 2–3 hours. Therefore, infants born less than 1 hour or more than 4 hours after a single dose of narcotic is administered to the mother usually show little or no effects. Since alphaprodine exerts its analgesic effect more rapidly than morphine or meperidine, it probably has a depressant effect on the fetus earlier. Even though its duration of action in the mother is shorter than these other drugs, however, it is possible that the fetal depressant effects may be of a duration similar to the others. If neonatal respiratory depression occurs in an alphaprodine-exposed newborn, naloxone should be immediately administered to the baby.

Petrie and associates reported that administration of alphaprodine, 20 mg given intravenously over 2 minutes, was followed by a statistically significant decrease in fetal heart rate variability in 10 of 14 (71%) patients studied. Both short-term and long-term variability were effected; these indices demonstrated a return toward normal values at 25 and 30 minutes, respectively.

After giving 40–60 mg alphaprodine intramuscularly to women in labor at 36 weeks gestation or later, Gray and colleagues noted that sinusoidal fetal heart rate patterns developed in 17 of 40 (42.5%) patients. This pattern appeared approximately 20 minutes following administration of the drug and persisted for about 60 minutes. In this study, 15 of the 17 babies with sinusoidal heart rates during labor had 1- and 5-minute Apgar scores of 7 or greater. The other 2 had low 1-minute Apgar scores that were directly associated with complications at delivery. The authors conclude that sinusoidal patterns developing during labor following the administration of alphaprodine are not associated with increased perinatal morbidity or mortality.

DOSAGE

Clinical trials in patients with postoperative pain have suggested the following approximate equivalent analgesic potencies.

Alphaprodine	Morphine Sulfate	Meperidine
30 mg	6 mg	50 mg
40 mg	8 mg	75 mg
50 mg	10 mg	100 mg

The optimum dosage range of alphaprodine for women in labor is 40–50 mg SC, 30–40 mg IM, or 15–20 mg IV. The onset of action is rapid, but the duration is less than that of other narcotics. Adequate analgesia usually only lasts 2–3 hours after SC administration and 1½–2 hours after IM or IV administration. Despite this, however, it is recommended that alphaprodine *not* be given more frequently than every 4 hours becuase of the potential for fetal depression in excess of observed analgesic effects in the mother. Bonica notes that the advantages of more rapid absorption and, therefore, more prompt analgesia over other narcotics when alphaprodine is given subcutaneously is lessened with intramuscular administration and eliminated when the drug is given intravenously.

ADVERSE EFFECTS

In equianalgesic doses the side effects of alphaprodine for the mother are very similar to those seen when morphine is used but are of shorter duration. It may cause respiratory depression, orthostatic hypotension, and urinary retention. Gastric emptying can be delayed, and constipation may result from a decrease in secretions and propulsive movements of the small and large bowel. Biliary tract smooth muscle tone is increased and spasm may result with large doses. Alphaprodine may cause less vomiting than some of the other narcotics.

MECHANISM OF ACTION

Alphaprodine, like the other narcotics, exerts its analgesic effect on the central nervous system. It produces analgesia, drowsiness, changes in mood, and mental clouding.

ABSORPTION AND BIOTRANSFORMATION

This drug is relatively ineffective orally but may be administered by subcutaneous, intramuscular, or intravenous routes. It is primarily metabolized in the liver. Like meperidine, alphaprodine probably undergoes hydrolysis and conjugation and is mainly excreted in the urine as the free drug or its glucuronide conjugate.

RECOMMENDED READING

Bonica, J. J. *Principles and Practice of Obstetric Analgesia and Anesthesia*. Philadelphia: F. A. Davis, 1967. Vol. 1, pp. 238–250.

Gillam, J. S., Hunter, G. W., Darner, C. B., and Thompson, G. R. Meperidine hydrochloride and alphaprodine hydrochloride as obstetric analgesic agents. *Am. J. Obstet. Gynecol.* 75:1105–1110, 1958.

Gray, J. H., Cudmore, D. W., Luther, E. R., Martin, T. R., and Gardner, A. J. Sinusoidal fetal heart rate pattern associated with alphaprodine administration. *Obstet. Gynecol.* 52:678–681, 1978.

Petrie, R. H., Yeh, S. Y., Murata, Y., Paul, R. H., Hon, E. H., Barron, B. A., and Johnson, R. J. The effect of drugs on fetal heart rate variability. *Am. J. Obstet. Gynecol.* 130:294–299, 1978.

(RLB)

Aminocaproic Acid (Amicar®)

INDICATIONS AND RECOMMENDATIONS

The use of aminocaproic acid (EACA) is contraindicated during pregnancy. It inhibits fibrinolysis and has been used in the treatment of excessive bleeding secondary to systemic and urinary hyperfibrinolysis. It has also been used in the treatment of acute exacerbations of hereditary angioneurotic edema.

EACA is a competitive inhibitor of plasminogen activators and to a lesser degree directly inhibits the action of plasmin. Any interference with plasmin activity results in a diminished capacity to hydrolyze fibrin, fibrinogen, and other clotting components. The thrombogenic capability of EACA is responsible for its most serious side effects, which include pulmonary emboli, intrapleural clot formation, and renal failure secondary to glomerular capillary thrombosis.

Patients with hereditary angioneurotic edema have a deficiency of Cl inhibitor, a substance that interferes with the activation of the first component of complement. Without this inhibitor, several components of the complement system combine to form a peptide that when cleaved by plasmin, increases the permeability of postcapillary venules and produces angioedema. It is by thus reducing plasminogenolysis that EACA produces beneficial effects in these patients. It should be noted that two cases of painful muscle necrosis have been reported in patients with hereditary angioneurotic edema whose conditions were treated with EACA.

Epsilon aminocaproic acid has been reported to be teratogenic in animals, but no congenital anomalies in humans have thus far been reported.

EACA should not be used during pregnancy unless a coagulopathy develops that can be proved to be caused by primary fibrinolysis. Hereditary angioneurotic edema tends to be a mild disease during pregnancy and investigators at the National Institutes of Health have recommended that EACA not be used to treat this condition in obstetric patients.

RECOMMENDED READING

Charytan, C., and Purtilo, D.   Glomerular capillary thrombosis and acute renal failure after epsilon aminocaproic acid therapy. *N. Engl. J. Med.* 280:1102–1104, 1969.

Frank, M. M., Gelfand, J. A., and Alling, D. W.   Epsilon aminocaproic acid for hereditary angioedema. *N. Engl. J. Med.* 296:1235–1236, 1977.

Johansson, S. A.   Acute right heart failure during treatment with epsilon aminocaproic acid (EACA). *Acta Med. Scand.* 182:331–334, 1967.

Korsan-Bengsten, K.   Extensive muscle necrosis after long-term treatment with aminocaproic acid in a case of hereditary periodic edema. *Acta Med. Scand.* 185:341–346, 1969.

McNicol, G. P.   Disordered fibrinolytic activity and its control. *Scott Med. J.* 7:266–274, 1974.

(BDH)

Aminoglycosides: Amikacin (Amikin®), Gentamicin (Garamycin®), Kanamycin (Kantrex®), Streptomycin, Tobramycin (Nebcin®)

INDICATIONS AND RECOMMENDATIONS

The aminoglycosides should be given during pregnancy only when serious gram-negative infections are suspected. Streptomycin has been used to treat enterococcal and *Streptococcus veridans* endocarditis, tuberculosis, plague, tularemia, and brucellosis. Kanamycin is used to treat serious aerobic gram-negative infections in which *Pseudomonas aeruginosa* is not suspected of being an etiological agent. Gentamicin, tobramycin, and amikacin are used to treat aerobic gram-negative infections, including those caused by *Pseudomonas aeruginosa.*

Gentamicin and kanamycin are preferable to tobramycin and amikacin because they have been more extensively studied. Tobramycin may be valuable in treating *Pseudomonas* infections in patients with cystic fibrosis.

SPECIAL CONSIDERATIONS IN PREGNANCY

There are no unusual effects on the mother during pregnancy. All of these drugs cross the placenta but have lower concentrations in fetal blood when tested at full term than in simultaneously determined maternal samples. Streptomycin and kanamycin have been noted to be associated with congenital deafness in the offspring of mothers taking this drug during pregnancy. It should therefore not be administered during the first trimester or in doses exceeding a total of 20 gm during the last half of pregnancy because of this potential danger. Ototoxicity has been reported with doses as low as 1 gm of streptomycin biweekly given for 8 weeks during the first trimester. Studies of effects of aminoglycoside administration during labor have not demonstrated toxicity to the fetus.

DOSAGE

Table 1 lists recommended dosages for the aminoglycosides.

ADVERSE EFFECTS

Streptomycin. Permanent vestibular eighth nerve damage may occur, as already noted. Paresthesias, rash, fever, pruritis, renal damage, and anaphylaxis are occasionally noted. Rarely, blood dyscrasias, optic neuritis, myocarditis, and hepatic necrosis may develop. Neuromuscular blockade and apnea have been reported with parenteral administration of the drug.

Nephrotoxicity may be increased when the drug is given with cephaloridine, cephalothin, or polymyxins. Ototoxicity may be increased by interaction with ethacrynic acid and neuromuscular blockade with curariform drugs.

Kanamycin. Occasionally, auditory eighth nerve damage will occur. This may remain undetected until after therapy has been stopped and can be irreversible. Renal damage, rash, and peripheral neuritis also have been noted. Parenteral or intraperitoneal administration may produce neuromuscular blockade or apnea.

Effects of drug interactions include increased nephrotoxicity with cephalosporins and polymyxins, ototoxicity with ethacrynic acid, and neuromuscular blockade with curariform drugs.

Table 1. Dosage Chart for Aminoglycosides

Drug	Oral Dosage	Oral Interval	Parenteral Dosage	Parenteral Interval (hours)	Usual Maximum Dose/Day	Dosage Interval for Creatinine Clearance (ml/min) 80–50	50–10	Less than 10
Streptomycin[a]			1–2 gm/day	q12	2 gm	24 hours	24–72 hours	72–96 hours
Kanamycin[a]			15 mg/kg/day	q8–12	1.5 gm	24 hours	24–72 hours	72–96 hours[b]
Gentamicin[a]			3–5 mg/kg/day	q8	5 mg/kg	12 hours[b]	12–36 hours[b]	48–72 hours[c]
Tobramycin[a]			3–5 mg/kg/day	q8	5 mg/kg	8–10 hours	10–36 hours	38–72 hours
Amikacin[a]			15 mg/kg/day	q8–12	1.5 gm	24 hours	24–72 hours	72–96 hours

Note: Oral neomycin and kanamycin are minimally absorbed from the gastrointestinal tract and therefore can be used for preoperative bowel sterilization.

[a] Administered parenterally only.
[b] Or calculate the interval between doses in hours as nine times the serum creatinine concentration in mg/100 ml.
[c] Or calculate the interval between doses in hours as eight times the serum creatinine concentration in mg/100 ml, or see nomogram in J. Hull, *Ann. Intern. Med.* 85:183, 1976.

Gentamicin. Occasionally, vestibular eighth nerve damage, rash, and renal impairment may occur. Rarely, auditory damage has been noted. Neuromuscular blockade and apnea may develop.

Effects of drug interactions include increased nephrotoxicity with cephalosporins and polymyxins, ototoxicity with ethacrynic acid, and neuromuscular blockade with curariform drugs.

Tobramycin and amikacin produce essentially the same side effects as gentamicin. They are newer drugs, however, and additional adverse sequelae may become evident in the future.

MECHANISM OF ACTION

The aminoglycoside antibiotics penetrate the cell wall and cytoplasmic membrane of susceptible microorganisms and act on the bacterial ribosomes. They bind to the ribosomes and cause a misreading of the microorganism's genetic code, which leads to the production of abnormal proteins and ultimately cell death.

ABSORPTION AND BIOTRANSFORMATION

These antibiotics are polycations, and their polarity is believed to be responsible for the pharmacokinetic properties common to the entire group. These include poor absorption after oral administration, poor penetration into the cerebrospinal fluid, and rapid excretion by the normal kidney. The aminoglycosides do not bind well to plasma proteins. Because their clearance is related to the glomerular filtration rate, dosage must be readjusted in the face of abnormal renal function.

RECOMMENDED READING

Handbook of Antimicrobial Therapy. The Medical Letter on Drugs and Therapeutics (Revised ed.), New Rochelle, N.Y.: The Medical Letter, 1978.

Robinson, G. C., and Cambon, K. G.   Hearing loss in infants of tuberculous mothers treated with streptomycin during pregnancy. *N. Engl. J. Med.* 271:949–951, 1964.

Weinstein, A. J., Gibbs, R. S., and Gallagher, M.   Placental transfer of clindamycin and gentamicin in term pregnancy. *Am. J. Obstet. Gynecol.* 124:688–691, 1976.

Yoshioka, H., Monma, T., and Matsuda, S.   Placental transfer of gentamicin. *J. Pediatr.* 80:121–123, 1972.

(GRD)

Amphetamines: Amphetamine sulfate (Benzedrine®), Dextroamphetamine sulfate (Dexedrine®)

INDICATIONS AND RECOMMENDATIONS

Amphetamines should not be used during pregnancy. These central sympathomimetic agents have been used as appetite suppressants, antifatigue agents, and in the treatment of narcolepsy. Although the data are conflicting, there are studies that show an increased incidence of cardiac defects and cleft palate following fetal exposure to amphetamine. At present, weight reduction and fatigue prevention are not valid indications for amphetamine therapy. Thus narcolepsy is the only clinical situation in which these drugs might be considered in the pregnant woman and methylphenidate is probably a better choice for this rare condition (see *Methylphenidate Hydrochloride*).

RECOMMENDED READING

Goodman, L. S., and Gilman, A. *The Pharmacological Basis of Therapeutics* (5th ed.). New York: Macmillan, 1975. Pp. 496–499.

Goodner, D. M. Teratology for the obstetrician. *Clin. Obstet. Gynecol.* 18:245–263, 1975.

Milkovich, L., and vandenBerg, B. J. Effects of antenatal exposure to anorectic drugs. *Am. J. Obstet. Gynecol.* 129:637–642, 1977.

(DRC)

Amphotericin B (Fungizone®)

INDICATIONS AND RECOMMENDATIONS

The use of amphotericin B during pregnancy should be limited to the treatment of life-threatening fungal infections such as cryptococcosis, blastomycosis, coccidiomycosis, histoplasmosis, mucormycosis, aspergillosis, and disseminated candidiasis. The safety of this drug during pregnancy has not been established. Patients receiving amphotericin B should be hospitalized and their renal function monitored at least once a week.

SPECIAL CONSIDERATIONS IN PREGNANCY

A study of teratogenic effects in mammals showed no developmental toxicity with amphotericin B. The literature describes 6 pregnancies during which the mother received amphotericin B: one pregnancy ended in a spontaneous abortion, one baby was small for gestational age and premature (the pregnancy was complicated by toxemia), one baby was born prematurely due to antepartum hemorrhage, and three pregnancies proceeded normally to full term. One full-term neonate had a transient rash that was attributed to amphotericin B.

DOSAGE

The recommended starting dose is 0.25 mg/kg/day with a gradual increase to 1 mg/kg/day as tolerance to the common side effects (chills and fever) develops. The maximum dose, to be given in severe infections, is 1.5 mg/kg/day. The usual duration of therapy is from 6 weeks to 4 months but may be shorter if side effects dictate discontinuation. The drug is administered intravenously in a concentration of 0.1 mg/ml over 4 to 6 hours. Because of the long plasma half-life, alternate-day dosing is feasible.

ADVERSE EFFECTS

Amphotericin B can potentially produce multiple toxicities. Nephrotoxicity, including hypokalemia, renal tubular acidosis, and abnormal urine sediment, is seen in over 80% of patients receiving this drug. The severity of renal impairment is dose-related, generally not reaching clinical significance unless the cumulative dose is 4 gm. Mild manifestations are reversible with cessation of therapy. Chills and fever (up to 40°C) are observed in upwards of 50% of patients at the time of initial intravenous injections. Vomiting, anorexia, headache, anemia, and phlebitis have all been reported. Hypersensitivity reactions have included anaphylaxis, thrombocytopenia, flushing, generalized pain, and convulsions.

ABSORPTION AND BIOTRANSFORMATION

Amphotericin B is poorly absorbed from the gastrointestinal tract and is therefore given intravenously for treatment of systemic infections. The plasma half-life is 24 hours. A small fraction of the dose appears in the urine, being detectable for as long as 7–8 weeks after therapy is discontinued. No abnormal accumulation is seen in patients with renal failure.

RECOMMENDED READING

Attkin, G. W., and Symonds, E. M. Cryptococcal meningitis in pregnancy treated with amphotericin B: A case report. *J. Obstet. Gynaecol. Br. Commonw.* 69:677–679, 1962.

Bindschadler, D. D., and Bennett, J. E.   A pharmacologic guide to the clinical use of amphotericin B. *J. Infect. Dis.* 120:427–436, 1969.

Feldman, R.   Cryptococcosis of the central nervous system—treated with amphotericin B during pregnancy. *Southern Med. J.* 52:1415, 1959.

Goodman, L. S., and Gilman, A.   *The Pharmacological Basis of Therapeutics* (5th ed.). New York: Macmillan, 1975. Pp. 1236–1238.

Kucus, A., and Bennet, N.   *The Use of Antibiotics* (2nd ed.). London: William Heinemann Medical Books, 1975. P. 873.

Philpot, C. R.   Cryptococcal meningitis in pregnancy. *Med. J. Aust.* 2:1005–1007, 1972.

Ruo, P.   A case of torulosis of the CNS during pregnancy. *Med. J. Aust.* 1:558–559, 1962.

Winn, W. A.   The use of amphotericin B in the treatment of coccidiodal disease. *Am. J. Med.* 27:617–635, 1959.

(TKM)

Anal Analgesics (Anugesic®, Anusol® suppository or ointment, Anusol-HC®)

INDICATIONS AND RECOMMENDATIONS

Anusol® suppositories or ointment are safe to use during pregnancy. These preparations are used for the symptomatic relief of pain or discomfort related to external or internal hemorrhoids, proctitis, cryptitis, fissures, and incomplete fistulas and for relief of local pain following anorectal surgery. The use of Anusol-HC® and Anugesic® are controversial and if used at all should be restricted to very specific situations.

SPECIAL CONSIDERATIONS IN PREGNANCY

Anusol-HC® contains 10.0 mg of hydrocortisone acetate and is often used for severe acute discomfort. Because topical steroids are absorbed systemically, this drug should be used during pregnancy with the same precautions as other steroid preparations.

DOSAGE

One Anusol® suppository may be inserted rectally in the morning, another at bedtime, and one following each bowel movement. Anusol® ointment can be applied externally, or inserted rectally with a plastic applicator. The ointment should be applied every 3–4 hours.

MECHANISM OF ACTION AND ADVERSE EFFECTS

Anusol® contains bismuth subgallate, bismuth resorcin, benzyl benzoate, peruvian balsam, and zinc oxide. The above combination provides a soothing, lubricating action on the mucous membranes, which relieves discomfort secondary to the passage of stool. No side effects have been noted.

Anugesic® contains pramoxine hydrochloride, which may cause a skin sensitivity reaction. This preparation therefore should be used with caution.

RECOMMENDED READING

Gerbie, A. B., and Sciarra, J. J. *Gynecology and Obstetrics.* Hagerstown, Md.: Harper & Row, 1978. Vol. 2. Ch 12:8.
Physician's Desk Reference (33rd ed.) Oradell, N.J.: Medical Economics Company, 1979. Pp. 1809–1810.

(GRD)

Antacids (over-the-counter): Aluminum hydroxide, Calcium carbonate, Magnesium compounds, Sodium bicarbonate

Many over-the-counter preparations include a combination of gastric antacids. The different components of these preparations will be described separately below.

One retrospective study suggested an association between the administration of aluminum hydroxide, calcium carbonate, and magnesium compound antacids during the first 56 days of gestation and the occurrence of major and minor congenital anomalies. It should be noted, however, that this was a heterogeneous group of anomalies. It was found that 5.9% of 458 mothers giving birth to anomalous babies took antacids during the first trimester, while 2.6% of 911 mothers of normal babies took these drugs. No causality can be inferred, and no substantiating data have followed.

Aluminum Hydroxide

INDICATIONS AND RECOMMENDATIONS

Aluminum hydroxide is safe to use during pregnancy in the last two trimesters. It is used to neutralize gastric acid and in the treatment of phosphate nephrolithiasis.

SPECIAL CONSIDERATIONS IN PREGNANCY

Some studies have shown increased deep tendon reflexes, hypomagnesemia, and possibly hypercalcemia in fetuses whose mothers were chronic users of aluminum hydroxide.

DOSAGE

Aluminum hydroxide comes in tablets containing 300 to 600 mg. A 600 mg dose will neutralize 2–10 mEq of acid in 30 minutes.

ADVERSE EFFECTS

Side effects of aluminum hydroxide include constipation; transient hypophosphatemia and hypophosphaturia; phosphate depletion syndrome with chronic use; increased calcium absorption, possibly leading to hypercalcemia and hypercalciuria; and hypomagnesemia. Aluminum hydroxide will decrease the absorption of tetracycline, chlorpromazine, acetylsalicylic acid, anticholinergic agents, pentobarbital, and sulfadiazine. The absorption of penicillin and pseudoephedrine are increased. There is a slight decrease in the absorption of amino acids, ascorbic acid, vitamin A, and glucose.

MECHANISM OF ACTION

Aluminum hydroxide reacts with hydrochloric acid in the stomach to form aluminum chloride. Nonabsorbed aluminum hydroxide is converted to insoluble aluminum phosphate in the gastrointestinal tract, making this a useful substance in the treatment of phosphate nephrolithiasis.

ABSORPTION AND BIOTRANSFORMATION

Between 17% and 31% of an oral dose of aluminum hydroxide may be recovered in the urine.

Calcium Carbonate

INDICATIONS AND RECOMMENDATIONS

Calcium carbonate is safe to use during pregnancy in the last two trimesters as long as chronic high doses are avoided. It is used to neutralize acid in the stomach.

SPECIAL CONSIDERATIONS IN PREGNANCY

Fetal hypomagnesemia, increased deep tendon reflexes, and increased muscle tone have been reported.

DOSAGE

The average dose of calcium carbonate is 1,000 mg; this will neutralize 13 mEq of acid in 30 minutes.

ADVERSE EFFECTS

Side effects include constipation, nausea, and belching. In predisposed persons, hypercalciuria with nephrolithiasis and azotemia may occur. Patients taking calcium carbonate for the treatment of ulcer disease may note "rebound" aggravation of their ulcer symptoms. In the milk-alkali syndrome, caused by the excessive intake of milk and/or soluble alkali, there is mild alkalosis, hypercalcemia, band keratopathy, distaste for food, nausea, vomiting, headache, and weakness. It is generally reversible after the calcium carbonate is discontinued.

MECHANISM OF ACTION

Calcium carbonate reacts with hydrochloric acid in the stomach to form calcium chloride, carbon dioxide, and water.

ABSORPTION AND BIOTRANSFORMATION

Calcium carbonate is absorbed at a rate of 10% to 15% by healthy individuals and 10% to 35% by persons with peptic ulcer disease. A transitory hypercalcemia is noted after an oral dose of calcium carbonate, but this effect is less marked if it is taken chronically by a person with normal renal function.

Magnesium Compounds

INDICATIONS AND RECOMMENDATIONS

Magnesium trisilicate, magnesium carbonate, and magnesium hydroxide are safe to use during pregnancy in the last two trimesters as long as chronic high doses are avoided. They are used to neutralize acid in the stomach.

SPECIAL CONSIDERATIONS IN PREGNANCY

Neonatal hypermagnesemia with drowsiness, decreased muscle tone, respiratory distress, and cardiovascular impairment have been reported in newborns exposed in utero to chronic high maternal magnesium levels. Silicaceous nephrolithiasis has also been reported in newborns whose mothers were chronic magnesium trisilicate takers.

DOSAGE

Magnesium trisilicate is taken as 500 mg tablets. The usual dose is 2 tablets, chewed thoroughly. This dose should neutralize 13–17 mEq of acid in 30 minutes. Magnesium hydroxide can be taken as a 310 mg tablet (neutralizes 10.7 mEq of acid) or as an 8% aqueous suspension (milk of magnesia); the usual dose is 5 ml, neutralizing 13.5 mEq of acid. When given in 15–30 ml doses, it is used as a cathartic.

ADVERSE EFFECTS

In patients with renal insufficiency, the magnesium compounds may cause hypermagnesemia with its associated muscle weakness and hypotonia, sedation, confusion, and in some cases, cardiovascular effects such as complete heart block. These compounds also may augment the absorption of warfarin compounds but decrease the absorption of barbiturates and weakly basic drugs such as quinidine. Chronic ingestion of magnesium trisilicate has been reported to result in formation of silicaceous stones in the urinary tract. Magnesium hydroxide acts as a cathartic when ingested in high doses.

MECHANISM OF ACTION

Magnesium trisilicate reacts with hydrochloric acid to form silicon dioxide and magnesium. The former substance, a gelatinous compound, may provide an adherent coating to an ulcer crater. Magnesium hydroxide (milk of magnesia 8%) reacts with hydrochloric acid to form magnesium chloride. Magnesium carbonate reacts with hydrochloric acid to form carbon dioxide and magnesium chloride.

ABSORPTION AND BIOTRANSFORMATION

Approximately 5% of the magnesium in magnesium trisilicate is absorbed. In both magnesium hydroxide and magnesium carbonate 5%–10% of the magnesium is absorbed.

Sodium Bicarbonate

INDICATIONS AND RECOMMENDATIONS

The use of sodium bicarbonate is relatively contraindicated during pregnancy because other therapeutic agents are preferable. It is used to neutralize stomach acid but is absorbed systemically (unlike most of the other antacid agents). The systemic absorption leads to a short duration of action, with a resultant rebound increase in symptoms. Chronic use also leads to systemic alkalosis. The sodium load that is absorbed can also cause edema and weight gain. For these reasons, it is recommended that other, less systemically active agents be used if antacid therapy is felt to be necessary.

RECOMMENDED READING

Goodman, L. S., and Gilman, A. *The Pharmacological Basis of Therapeutics* (5th ed.). New York: Macmillan, 1975. Pp. 960–966.

Nelson, M. M., and Forfar, J. O. Associations between drugs administered during pregnancy and congenital abnormalities of the fetus. *Br. Med. J.* 1:523–527, 1971.

Schenkel, B., and Vorherr, H. Non-prescription drugs during pregnancy: Potential teratogenic and toxic effects upon embryo and fetus. *J. Reprod. Med.* 12:27–45, 1974.

(RAC)

Antihistamines (over-the-counter): Brompheniramine, Chlorpheniramine, Cyclizine, Doxylamine, Meclizine, Phenindamine, Pheniramine, Pyrilamine

INDICATIONS AND RECOMMENDATIONS

Antihistamines in pregnancy should be limited to their use in the treatment of allergic symptoms, the prophylaxis of motion sickness, and as sedatives. The antihistamine compounds available in over-the-counter (OTC) preparations, with the exception of brompheniramine, have not been implicated as having deleterious effects in the pregnant woman or fetus. As with any drug, however, antihistamines should be used only when absolutely necessary during pregnancy. Chlorpheniramine does not appear to have teratogenic effects at recommended doses; however, no prospective studies are available. These drugs are not recommended for use by lactating women.

SPECIAL CONSIDERATIONS IN PREGNANCY

A large-scale study of drugs that could possibly have a teratogenic effect if taken during pregnancy included the following antihistamines available in OTC preparations: chlorpheniramine, pheniramine, and brompheniramine. Of these, only with brompheniramine was there a statistically significant increased risk of teratogenicity. Animal studies have implicated meclizine and cyclizine as teratogenic agents. Large-scale studies in humans, however, have not shown an increased incidence of death or malformations in children of women who used any of these drugs during pregnancy. When, as is usual, they are found in combination products, the potential effects of all ingredients must be considered.

Due to its anticholinergic properties, chlorpheniramine may inhibit lactation. In addition, small amounts may be secreted into breast milk. This drug and all antihistamines, therefore, should be avoided by the lactating mother.

DOSAGE

The dosage amount of any of these antihistamines varies with the particular preparation in which it is found. They are often found combined with other ingredients.

ADVERSE EFFECTS

Side effects of antihistamines are most commonly anticholinergic in nature and include dryness of the mouth, difficulty in voiding, and, rarely, impotence. Dizziness, lassitude, incoordination, fatigue, blurred vision, and nervousness also occur. Digestive tract effects include anorexia, nausea, vomiting, constipation, and diarrhea, all of which may be avoided by taking the drug with meals. Leukopenia and agranulocytosis are rarely seen. Toxic doses result in hallucinations, ataxia, athetosis, and convulsions. Death may result from cardiorespiratory collapse.

MECHANISM OF ACTION

These compounds act by competitive antagonism to prevent histamine from exerting its vasodilatory and bronchoconstrictive effects. They are effective in suppressing the symptoms of seasonal rhinitis but are less effective in the treatment of perennial rhinitis. They may also be effective in the treatment of certain allergic dermatoses. Antihistamines also have central effects that account for their sedative properties and their efficacy in the prevention of motion sickness.

ABSORPTION AND BIOTRANSFORMATION

The pharmacokinetics of these drugs are not well known. They are well absorbed from the gastrointestinal tract. As a group, they seem to be metabolized in the liver with little if any being excreted unchanged in the urine.

RECOMMENDED READING

Goodman, L. S., and Gilman, A. *The Pharmacological Basis of Therapeutics* (5th ed.). New York: Macmillan 1975. Pp. 603–611.

Greenberger, P., and Patterson, R.   Safety of therapy for allergic symptoms during pregnancy. *Ann. Intern. Med.* 89:234–237, 1978.

Heinonen, O. P., Slone, D., and Shapiro, S. *Birth Defects and Drugs in Pregnancy*. Littleton, Mass.: Publishing Sciences Group, 1977. Pp. 322–334.

(RAC)

Atropine

INDICATIONS AND RECOMMENDATIONS

During pregnancy parenteral atropine should be limited to its use as a preanesthetic agent in surgical patients to reduce salivation and bronchial secretions. It diminishes beat-to-beat heart rate variability and may mask the effects of vagal stimulation on the fetal heart. The intrapartum administration of atropine for the treatment of fetal bradycardia is controversial, but most perinatologists feel that it currently has no role in this setting.

Ophthalmic solutions for topical administration may be used to produce mydriasis and cycloplegia for refraction and in the treatment of inflammatory conditions of the uveal tract. Systemic absorption can be minimized by compressing the lacrimal sac during and for 1 minute following instillation of the drops.

The use of belladonna alkaloids in over-the-counter preparations is discussed under *Belladonna Alkaloids*.

SPECIAL CONSIDERATIONS IN PREGNANCY

Atropine crosses the placenta and is secreted in breast milk; 93% of the maternal serum concentration has been found in umbilical vein blood within 5 minutes of the time the drug was injected into the maternal circulation. Fetal lamb studies have shown that atropine inhibits fetal bradycardia and may increase carotid and cerebral blood flow. In the human fetus atropine is known to diminish beat-to-beat variability and to mask variable fetal heart rate decelerations.

DOSAGE

The usual parenteral dose is 0.5–1 mg. The ophthalmic dose is 1–2 drops of a 0.5%, 1%, 2%, or 3% solution instilled 1 hour before refraction or up to three times a day for treatment of uveitis.

ADVERSE EFFECTS

Annoying anticholinergic effects include dryness of mucous membranes, thirst, and constipation. In larger doses slurred speech and blurred vision may occur. Overdosage may produce ataxia, excitement, disorientation, hallucinations, delirium, coma, high fever, and antidiuresis.

MECHANISM OF ACTION

The principle action of atropine occurs as a competitive antagonism of acetylcholine at muscarinic sites. It also has a direct effect on the medulla and higher cerebral centers.

Atropine-induced parasympathetic block may be preceded by a transient phase of mild stimulation. This is probably a result of central vagal stimulation by doses too small to block peripheral muscarinic receptors. With average clinical doses the heart rate may be minimally slowed. Larger doses, however, cause progressively increasing tachycardia by blocking vagal effects on the pacemaker in the sinoatrial node. Atropine decreases intestinal motility by blocking extrinsic parasympathetic nervous control as well as that of intramural nerve plexuses. Mydriasis and cycloplegia occur because atropine blocks the responses of the sphincter muscle of the iris and the ciliary muscle of the lens to cholinergic stimulation. In addition, the secretory activity of exocrine glands is decreased.

ABSORPTION AND BIOTRANSFORMATION

Atropine is usually administered parenterally, but it is well absorbed from all mucosal surfaces. Only limited absorption occurs from the eye, but any portion of a dose that traverses the nasolacrimal duct into the pharynx will be absorbed. Atropine is primarily hydrolyzed in the liver. Most of the drug is excreted in the urine within the first 12 hours, 13%–50% being unchanged and the remainder appearing as metabolites.

RECOMMENDED READING

Cohn, H. E., Piasecki, G. J., and Jackson, B. T. The effect of atropine blockade on the fetal cardiovascular response to hypoxemia. *Gynecol. Invest.* 7:57, 1976.

Goodlin, R. C. Inappropriate fetal bradycardia. *Obstet. Gynecol.* 48:117–122, 1976.

Goodlin, R. C., and Haesslein, H. Fetal reacting bradycardia. *Am. J. Obstet. Gynecol.* 129:845–856, 1977.

Goodman, L. S., and Gilman, A. *The Pharmacological Basis of Therapeutics* (5th ed.). New York: Macmillan, 1975. Pp. 515–523.

Ikenoue, T., Quilligan, E. J., and Murata, Y. Circulatory response to atropine in sheep fetus. *Am. J. Obstet. Gynecol.* 126:253–260, 1976.

Kivado, I., and Saari Roski, S. Placental transmission of atropine at full term pregnancy. *Br. J. Anaesth.* 49:1017–1021, 1977.

(TKM)

Beclomethasone (Vanceril®)

INDICATIONS AND RECOMMENDATIONS

Beclomethasone may be used for the pregnant woman who needs steroids to control her bronchospasm and in whom systemic steroid therapy may not be necessary. It is an aerosol glucocorticoid compound that has been used in patients who have failed to respond to bronchodilators and cromolyn sodium. It should be appreciated that the effect of beclomethasone on the fetus is presently unknown.

SPECIAL CONSIDERATIONS IN PREGNANCY

There are no well-controlled studies relating to fetal risk when mothers use this drug. It is unknown if the drug crosses the human placenta or is secreted into breast milk. Animal studies involving systemic glucocorticosteroids have suggested an increase in early fetal loss, cleft palate, and other malformations.

DOSAGE

The recommended dose is two inhalations (50 μg per inhalation) every 6–8 hours, with the maximal recommended dose 1,000 μg/day. This dosage did not produce suppression of early morning cortisol concentration in adult volunteers. If a patient is to be switched from chronic oral systemic corticosteroids to beclomethasone, the aerosol should be used along with the systemic steroid. After 2 weeks the steroid dosage can be reduced by 2.5 mg prednisone or equivalent every 2 weeks.

ADVERSE EFFECTS

Unlike systemic steroids, inhaled beclomethasone has minimal systemic effects. In conventional doses, it produces little or no suppression of the pituitary-adrenal axis. Side effects include hoarseness, oral candidiasis, and an increased incidence of pulmonary infection.

MECHANISM OF ACTION

Although the mode of action of steroids in asthma remains unclear, their effects are probably multiple and are mediated mainly through their anti-inflammatory effect. In controlled trials inhaled beclomethasone has been shown to be as effective as oral prednisone in controlling the symptoms of mild to moderate asthma in those asthmatics who require long-term corticosteroid therapy.

The drug is not useful in an acute asthmatic attack since bronchospasm may prevent its distribution to more distal airways.

ABSORPTION AND BIOTRANSFORMATION

Beclomethasone is administered by a metered-dose oral unit. The drug is deposited in the mouth, nasal mucosa, trachea, bronchi, and lung tissue; a significant amount is swallowed. Systemic absorption does occur. The principal route of elimination of the drug and its metabolites is via the feces. Hypersensitivity to the drug and its propellant (trichlorofluoromethane and dichlorofluoromethane) has been reported.

RECOMMENDED READING

Choo-Kang, Y. F. J., Cooper, J., Tribe, A. E., and Grant, I. W. Beclomethasone dipropionate by inhalation in the treatment of airways obstruction. *Br. J. Dis. Chest* 66:101–106, 1972.

Clark, T. J. H. Effect of beclomethasone dipropionate delivered by aerosol in patients with asthma. *Lancet* 1:1361–1364, 1972.

Lal, S., Harris, D. M., Bhala, K. K., Singhal, S. N., and Butler, A. G. Comparison of beclomethasone dipropionate aerosol and prednisone in reversible airway obstruction. *Br. Med. J.* 3:314–317, 1972.

Martin, L. E., Tanner, R. J. N., Clark, T. J. H., and Cochrane, G. M. Absorption and metabolism of orally administered beclomethasone dipropionate. *Clin. Pharmacol. Ther.* 15:267–275, 1974.

Simon, G. The place of new aerosol steroid beclomethasone dipropionate in the management of childhood asthma. *Pediatr. Clin. North Am.* 22:147–155, 1975.

(RJR)

Belladonna Alkaloids (over-the-counter): Atropine, Homatropine, Scopolamine

INDICATIONS AND RECOMMENDATIONS

Belladonna alkaloids and their quaternary ammonium derivatives are present in a variety of over-the-counter (OTC) antidiarrheal and sedative products. They are usually combined with adsorbents for the treatment of diarrhea, and antihistamines and analgesics for use as sedatives. As the belladonna alkaloids are not present in recognized therapeutic doses in OTC antidiarrheal preparations, and since other nonabsorbable agents are available, their use for this purpose during pregnancy is not necessary. Products containing scopolamine in therapeutic doses appear to be safe when used in the treatment of insomnia in pregnancy before the onset of labor.

SPECIAL CONSIDERATIONS IN PREGNANCY

The use of atropine near term has been associated with decreased beat-to-beat heart rate variability in the fetus. This phenomenon has been seen primarily with large-dose parenteral use. Small amounts of atropine are secreted in breast milk. When bromides are also contained in compounds, acneiform rash, hypotonia and lethargy, irritability, high-pitched cry, and difficulty feeding have been reported in the newborn.

DOSAGE

The usual doses of the belladonna alkaloids available in OTC medications are quite small. Scopolamine is found in doses of 0.083–0.5 mg in combination with other ingredients in OTC sedatives. The total dose of all belladonna alkaloids in the usual antidiarrheal compound is about 0.13 mg/30 ml.

ADVERSE EFFECTS

The most common side effect of these agents is dryness of the mouth and throat. Other anticholinergic effects such as blurred vision, photophobia, and urinary retention are uncommon at the dosage provided in OTC preparations. Scopolamine may disrupt the sleep cycle by decreasing rapid eye movement (REM) time. When it is discontinued after several days of use, a rebound in REM occurs, resulting in nightmares, insomnia, and the feeling of having slept badly. This effect is not usual at the doses present in most OTC preparations, but it may be experienced by patients who use these preparations chronically or who exceed recommended dosages.

The belladonna alkaloids are rapidly absorbed into the bloodstream and are distributed throughout the body. Elimination varies with the individual agent. The majority of the compounds are metabolized but 13%–50% of atropine and 1% of scopolamine are excreted in the urine unchanged.

MECHANISM OF ACTION

These antimuscarinic agents competitively inhibit acetylcholine at the receptor site of the effector organ. When used in doses equivalent to 0.6–1 mg of atropine sulfate, belladonna alkaloids are effective in the treatment of diarrhea due to increased intestinal tone and peristalsis. However, most OTC antidiarrheal agents containing belladonna alkaloids contain less than this recognized effective dose.

When a sedative effect is the primary one required, scopolamine is the agent used. It acts as a hypnotic by depressing the cerebral cortex. Therapeutic doses produce drowsiness, euphoria, fatigue, and dreamless sleep.

RECOMMENDED READING

Goodman, L. S., and Gilman, A. *The Pharmacological Basis of Therapeutics* (5th ed.). New York: Macmillan, 1975. Pp. 518–523, 528–530.

Nelson, M. M., and Forfar, J. O. Associations between drugs administered during pregnancy and congenital abnormalities of the fetus. *Br. Med. J.* 1:523–527, 1971.

Schenkel, B., and Vorherr, H. Non-prescription drugs during pregnancy: Potential teratogenic and toxic effects upon embryo and fetus. *J. Reprod. Med.* 12:27–45, 1974.

(RAC)

Bromocriptine (Parlodel®)

INDICATIONS AND RECOMMENDATIONS

Bromocriptine is contraindicated during pregnancy. It is used primarily for the induction of ovulation in women with galactorrhea-amenorrhea syndromes. It may have some value in the treatment of anovulation in general, especially in patients with corpus luteum insufficiency. It is used in the treatment of galactorrhea and also has a potential application as a lactation-suppressing agent.

No data exist on the physiological effect of bromocriptine on the fetus. Although many patients have inadvertently taken this drug in early pregnancy, there is no evidence that it is associated with teratogenic effects.

The drug is contraindicated in pregnancy because once pregnancy has occurred there is no further need for induction of ovulation. Bromocriptine is an effective suppressant of breast milk production and may be used in the postpartum period for this purpose.

RECOMMENDED READING

Mroueh, A. M., and Siler-Khodr, T. M. Bromocryptine therapy in cases of amenorrhea-galactorrhea. *Am. J. Obstet. Gynecol.* 127:291–298, 1977.

Tolis, G., and Naftolin, F. Induction of menstruation with bromocryptine in patients with euprolactinemic amenorrhea. *Am. J. Obstet. Gynecol.* 126:426–429, 1976.

Wiebe, R. H. Treatment of functional amenorrhea-galactorrhea with 2-bromoergocryptine. *Fertil. Steril.* 28:426–433, 1977.

(AHD)

Bulk Forming Agents (over-the-counter): Agar, Bran, Methylcellulose, Psyllium, Tragacanth

INDICATIONS AND RECOMMENDATIONS

Bulk forming agents are safe to use during pregnancy. The over-the-counter drugs listed above are used as stool softeners in people with constipation, hemorrhoids, anorectal disorders, hernias, and cardiovascular disease.

SPECIAL CONSIDERATIONS IN PREGNANCY

There are no maternal effects unique to pregnancy.

DOSAGE

Methylcellulose and carboxymethylcellulose are supplied as a 500 mg powder, tablet, or capsule. The dose is 1–6 gm/day taken one to four times a day, each dose taken with 1–2 glasses of water. Onset of action is 1–2 days.

Psyllium preparations from the plantain seed are powders. One to two teaspoons of powder are mixed in water and taken one to three times a day.

Agar is usually mixed with psyllium or cathartics and 4–16 gm are taken daily.

Tragacanth is available in many preparations in a variety of dosages.

Bran contains 20% indigestible cellulose and is generally taken with cereal.

ADVERSE EFFECTS

With the exception of the psyllium preparations, none of these bulk forming laxatives is significantly absorbed and thus no systemic effects occur. Psyllium preparations are absorbed to some degree and have been shown to decrease plasma cholesterol levels by interfering with absorption of bile acids. Bulk forming laxatives may increase flatulence, and if taken with inadequate water intestinal obstruction may occur.

MECHANISM OF ACTION

These agents, which include methylcellulose and carboxymethyl-cellulose, psyllium preparations, agar, tragacanth, and bran, all swell when in contact with water, forming a mass that promotes peristalsis, decreases transit time, and keeps the feces soft.

RECOMMENDED READING

Goodman, L. S., and Gilman, A. *The Pharmacological Basis of Therapeutics* (5th ed.). New York: Macmillan, 1975. Pp. 946–947, 978–980.

Nelson, M. M., and Forfar, J. O. Associations between drugs administered during pregnancy and congenital abnormalities of the fetus. *Br. Med. J.* 1:523–527, 1971.

Schenkel, B., and Vorherr, H. Non-prescription drugs during pregnancy: Potential teratogenic and toxic effects upon embryo and fetus. *J. Reprod. Med.* 12:27–45, 1974.

(RAC)

Camphor (over-the-counter)

INDICATIONS AND RECOMMENDATIONS

Camphor is safe to use during pregnancy. This drug is applied topically and produces a local anesthetic and antipruritic effect. When taken orally, it can relieve or prevent flatulence, and it is an ingredient in paregoric.

SPECIAL CONSIDERATIONS IN PREGNANCY

There are no maternal effects unique to pregnancy. It is theoretically possible for fetal convulsions to occur if large doses are taken systemically.

ADVERSE EFFECTS

Camphor is a rubefacient when rubbed on the skin. If not vigorously applied, however, it may cause a feeling of coolness.

When taken systemically camphor may stimulate the central nervous system. It does not selectively stimulate respiration and has very little effect on the circulation. If children ingest large amounts of solid camphor, convulsions can occur. In small oral doses this drug produces a sensation of warmth and comfort in the stomach. It may, however, cause nausea and vomiting in larger doses.

RECOMMENDED READING

Goodman, L. S., and Gilman, A. *The Pharmacological Basis of Therapeutics* (5th ed.). New York: Macmillan, 1975. Pp. 951–952.

Nelson, M. M., and Forfar, J. O. Associations between drugs administered during pregnancy and congenital abnormalities of the fetus. *Br. Med. J.* 1:523–527, 1971.

Schenkel, B., and Vorherr, H. Non-prescription drugs during pregnancy: Potential teratogenic and toxic effects upon embryo and fetus. *J. Reprod. Med.* 12:27–45, 1974.

(RAC)

Candicidin (Candeptin®)

INDICATIONS AND RECOMMENDATIONS

Candicidin vaginal ointment and tablets are safe to use during pregnancy for the treatment of candidal vaginitis. These preparations should not be applied vaginally when membranes are ruptured.

SPECIAL CONSIDERATIONS IN PREGNANCY

No teratogenic effects have been reported with intravaginal candicidin. Microbiological cure rates between 59% and 100% have been reported. Pregnant patients appear to require a longer duration of therapy or multiple treatment courses for a complete clinical and microbiological cure.

DOSAGE

Candicidin is available as a vaginal ointment and in vaginal tablet form. The recommended dosage is the contents of one applicator or one tablet inserted high into the vagina, twice daily, for 14 days.

MECHANISM OF ACTION

Candicidin is a polyene antibiotic that alters yeast membrane permeability, allowing leakage of essential metabolic substrates.

ABSORPTION AND BIOTRANSFORMATION

Candicidin is not absorbed to a significant extent through the vaginal mucosa.

RECOMMENDED READING

Bodey, G. P., Adachi, L., and Jones, V. Effects of candicidin on fungal flora of gastrointestinal tract. *Curr. Ther. Res.* 16:207–213, 1974.

Hammond, G. M., and Kliger, B. N.   Mode of action of polyene antibiotic candicidin: Binding factors in wall of *Candida albicans. Antimicrob. Agents Chemother.* 9:561–568, 1976.

Melges, F. J.   A new antifungal antibiotic? *Obstet. Gynecol.* 24:921–923, 1964.

Morese, K. N.   Candicidin tablets and ointment in treatment of candidal vaginitis. *N.Y. State J. Med.* 75:1443–1445, 1975.

Vartiainen, E., and Tervila, L.   Use of Candeptin® for treatment of moniliasis. *Acta Obstet. Gynecol. Scand.* 49(Suppl):2:21–24, 1970.

(TKM)

Carbamazepine (Tegretol®)

INDICATIONS AND RECOMMENDATIONS

The use of carbamazepine during pregnancy should be limited to the treatment of trigeminal neuralgia, intractable hiccoughs, and seizures refractory to therapy with established agents. It is a second-line drug for the treatment of grand mal, psychomotor, and focal seizures. The risk of taking carbamazepine in pregnancy is unknown. If this drug is administered, it is imperative that plasma levels be monitored and hematological, hepatic, renal, and cardiovascular parameters be closely followed.

SPECIAL CONSIDERATIONS IN PREGNANCY

Teratogenesis has been demonstrated in rats and mice but has not yet been documented in humans. Carbamazepine is excreted in breast milk in very small amounts.

DOSAGE

The initial dose is 100 mg by mouth bid; dosage may be increased to as high as 1,200 mg per day to achieve seizure control. The therapeutic plasma level has been proposed as 6–8 μg/ml.

ADVERSE EFFECTS

Side effects have been related to plasma levels of the drug and are first seen at a concentration of 1.5 μg/ml. In 50% of patients side effects are noted at 8.5–10 μg/ml. Commonly observed problems include diplopia, dysarthria, nystagmus, drowsiness, fatigue, ataxia, headache, and gastrointestinal complaints. Skin rash occurs in 3% of patients. Major side effects are hematological (leukopenia, aplastic anemia, thrombocytopenia, purpura); cardiovascular (left ventricular failure, cardiovascular collapse, with fatalities reported); renal (acute oliguria with hypertension); hepatic (jaundice); and thrombophlebitis. In addition, photosensitivity, exfoliative dermatitis, and a lupus-like syndrome have been observed. Drug interactions with coumarin (increased metabolism) and phenytoin (decreased serum levels) have been described.

MECHANISM OF ACTION

Carbamazepine blocks posttetanic potentiation and appears to act selectively on areas of the brain frequently involved in epileptogenesis. Its therapeutic effect in trigeminal neuralgia is particularly related to the blockade of afferent synaptic transmission in the trigeminal nerve.

ABSORPTION AND BIOTRANSFORMATION

Carbamazepine is well absorbed orally, is highly protein bound, and is metabolized in the liver. The plasma half-life averages 1 to 2 days.

RECOMMENDED READING

Eadie, M. J., and Tyrer, J. H. *Anticonvulsant Therapy*. Edinburgh: Churchill-Livingstone, 1974.

Goodman, L. S., and Gilman, A. *The Pharmacological Basis of Therapeutics* (5th ed.). New York: Macmillan, 1975. Pp. 211–212.

Niebyl, J. R., Blake, D. A., Freeman, J. M., and Luff, R. D. Carbamazepine levels in pregnancy and lactation. *Obstet. Gynecol.* 53:139–140, 1979.

Tuchmann-Duplessis, H. *Drug Effects on the Fetus*. Sydney, Australia: Adis Press, 1975.

Woodbury, D. M., Penry, J. K., and Schmidt, R. P. *Antiepileptic Drugs*. New York: Raven Press, 1972.

(PHR)

Cathartics, Contact (over-the-counter)

Anthracene cathartics: Aloe, Cascara, Danthron, Senna

INDICATIONS AND RECOMMENDATIONS

With the exception of aloe, anthracene cathartics are safe to use during pregnancy. Despite their safety, however, attention to proper diet and exercise is preferable to dependence upon these agents. The anthracene cathartics include senna, cascara sagrada, and danthron. Aloe is contraindicated in pregnancy because it can cross the placenta and stimulate the fetal intestine, leading to the passage of meconium.

SPECIAL CONSIDERATIONS IN PREGNANCY

Aloe should not be used in pregnancy for the above-mentioned reason.

DOSAGE

Senna is taken in a 2 gm dose with results in 6 hours. Fluid extract of cascara sagrada, 2.5 ml, will give results in 8 hours. Danthron causes stool-softening 6–8 hours after a 25–150 mg dose.

ADVERSE EFFECTS

Side effects include intestinal melanosis with prolonged use. This is reversible when the drug is discontinued.

MECHANISM OF ACTION

The anthracene cathartics act directly on the bowel wall to stimulate intestinal motility, which is primarily a large bowel effect. They are hydrolyzed by colonic bacteria with release of the active agent.

Castor Oil

INDICATIONS AND RECOMMENDATIONS

Castor oil is safe to use during pregnancy. It is used as a cathartic agent, most commonly when patients are to have x-rays of the kidney or colon, or both.

SPECIAL CONSIDERATIONS IN PREGNANCY

Although abdominal x-rays are relatively contraindicated during pregnancy, the use of castor oil in preparation for x-rays poses no special problems to the obstetrical patient.

DOSAGE

The usual dose is 15–30 ml by mouth on demand.

ADVERSE EFFECTS

The major problem with castor oil is its very unpleasant taste. There is also some evidence of potential cytotoxic effects on the small intestine.

MECHANISM OF ACTION

Castor oil is hydrolyzed in the small intestine to glycerol and ricinoleic acid, the latter of which stimulates motility of the small intestine.

Diphenylmethanes: Bisacodyl, Phenolphthalein

INDICATIONS AND RECOMMENDATIONS

Diphenylmethanes are safe to use during pregnancy. Despite their safety, however, attention to proper diet and exercise is preferable to dependence upon these agents. The diphenylmethanes include phenolphthalein and bisacodyl and are widely used in over-the-counter cathartic preparations.

SPECIAL CONSIDERATIONS IN PREGNANCY

There are no special considerations in pregnancy.

DOSAGE

Phenolphthalein is taken in a dose of 60–200 mg and acts in 6–8 hours. Bisacodyl is taken in a dose of 10–15 mg orally, acting in 6–8 hours, or as a 10 mg rectal suppository acting within 15–60 minutes.

ADVERSE EFFECTS

Side effects include cramps, mucous stools, and excessive fluid loss in the stools. Allergic skin reactions have been reported with phenolphthalein. Proctitis has been reported with bisacodyl.

MECHANISM OF ACTION

These drugs act mainly on the large intestine, stimulating peristalsis.

ABSORPTION AND BIOTRANSFORMATION

Although phenolphthalein is mainly excreted in the feces, up to 15% may be absorbed, conjugated, and excreted in the urine. Some is excreted in bowel. The urine or stools, or both, will be pink to red in color if the pH is alkaline.

Up to 5% of bisacodyl is absorbed and conjugated as a glucuronide appearing in the urine.

RECOMMENDED READING

Goodman, L. S., and Gilman, A. *The Pharmacological Basis of Therapeutics* (5th ed.). New York: Macmillan, 1975. Pp. 982–983.

Nelson, M. M., and Forfar, J. O. Associations between drugs administered during pregnancy and congenital abnormalities of the fetus. *Br. Med. J.* 1:523–527, 1971.

Schenkel, B., and Vorherr, H. Non-prescription drugs during pregnancy: Potential teratogenic and toxic effects upon embryo and fetus. *J. Reprod. Med.* 12:27–45, 1974.

(RAC)

Cathartics, Saline (over-the-counter): Magnesium salts, including milk of magnesia and epsom salt; sodium and potassium salts

INDICATIONS AND RECOMMENDATIONS

Saline cathartics, which include magnesium, sodium, and potassium salts, are safe to use during pregnancy. Their use, however, should be avoided in patients with significant cardiovascular disease or impairment of renal function. They are used for cathartic cleaning of the bowel prior to surgery and radiologic or proctological examination, in patients with functional constipation, and in those with constipation due to inadequate fluid intake or exercise.

SPECIAL CONSIDERATIONS IN PREGNANCY

There are no special considerations in pregnancy.

DOSAGE

Of the magnesium salts magnesium sulfate (epsom salt) is given in doses of 15–30 gm. It should be dissolved in fruit juice to overcome the objectionable taste. Magnesium citrate is available in a 10-ounce bottle of effervescent solution. The usual dose is 5–10 ounces. Some patients are nauseated by this preparation, and its action may be quite violent. Magnesium hydroxide is available in an 8% aqueous solution (milk of magnesia), and the usual dose is 8–30 ml. It also acts as an antacid.

The usual cathartic dose of the phosphate salts of sodium and potassium is from 4–20 gm. The onset of action for these preparations is 3 to 6 hours or less.

ADVERSE EFFECTS

There is little systemic effect except for the possibility of dehydration resulting from fluid loss in the feces; this occurs because they are so slowly absorbed that they retain water in the gastrointestinal tract and may even draw fluid into it. Congestive heart failure because of the salt load could occur in patients predisposed to this condition. Magnesium intoxication may occur in patients with impaired renal function.

RECOMMENDED READING

Goodman, L. S., and Gilman, A. *The Pharmacological Basis of Therapeutics* (5th ed.). New York: Macmillan, 1975. P. 980.

Nelson, M. M., and Forfar, J. O. Associations between drugs administered during pregnancy and congenital abnormalities of the fetus. *Br. Med. J.* 1:523–527, 1971.

Schenkel, B., and Vorherr, H. Non-prescription drugs during pregnancy: Potential teratogenic and toxic effects upon embryo and fetus. *J. Reprod. Med.* 12:27–45, 1974.

(RAC)

Cephalosporins: Cefaclor (Ceclor®) Cefadroxil (Duricef®), Cefamandole (Mandol®), Cefazolin (Ancef®, Kefzol®), Cefoxitin (Mefoxin®), Cephalexin (Keflex®), Cephaloridine (Loridine®), Cephalothin (Keflin®), Cephapirin (Cefadyl®), Cephradine (Anspor®, Velosef®)

INDICATIONS AND RECOMMENDATIONS

The cephalosporins are safe to use during pregnancy. These drugs are broad-spectrum antibiotics that have been extensively used during pregnancy because of their low potential for toxicity and clinical effectiveness. They are effective against infections caused by streptococci, *Staphylococcus aureus, Escherichia coli*, and *Klebsiella, Proteus, Salmonella*, and *Shigella* species. The following bacteria are relatively resistant to these drugs: enterococci, *Bacteroides fragilis, Enterobacter aerogenes, Serratia marcescens* and *Pseudomonas aeruginosa.*

Cefoxitin and cefamandole are recently marketed second-generation cephalosporins. Both are effective against *B. fragilis* strains while the first generation drugs are not. Until more experience is accumulated in pregnant women, however, other broad-spectrum antibiotics are recommended rather than these two agents.

SPECIAL CONSIDERATIONS IN PREGNANCY

There are no special maternal effects when these drugs are administered during pregnancy. They cross the placenta but no teratogenic effects have been reported to date. The presence of cefazolin in second trimester abortuses has been studied. The drug was found in fetal serum and urine as well as in amniotic fluid in concentrations lower than that found in maternal serum. It was not detected in the fetal brain, cerebrospinal fluid, lung, liver, or kidneys.

DOSAGE

Table 2 details recommended dosages.

ADVERSE EFFECTS

Side effects include thrombophlebitis with intravenous use and a serum sickness-like reaction with prolonged parenteral administration. Allergic reactions and gastrointestinal disturbances may occur. The incidence of hypersensitivity reactions to the cephalosporins is higher in patients who have shown an allergic reaction to penicillin. This is apparently related to sensitization to the beta-lactam ring common to both drugs. Controversy exists as to the incidence of cross-sensitivity to this drug. With the exception of patients who have had anaphylactic reactions to penicillin, however, cephalosporins are not contraindicated in patients with penicillin allergy.

Rarely, hemolytic anemia, hepatic dysfunction, blood dyscrasias, and renal damage (especially with cephaloridine) may occur. Toxic renal damage may be potentiated by the concurrent use of aminoglycosides, probenecid, or potent diuretics such as furosemide or ethacrynic acid.

MECHANISM OF ACTION

These drugs inhibit bacterial cell wall synthesis and are consequently bactericidal. The cephalosporins, like penicillin, contain a beta-lactam ring. They also have a dihydrothiazine ring with attached side chains that give the various compounds their individual properties.

Table 2. Dosage Chart for Cephalosporins

Drug	Oral Dosage (gm/day)	Oral Interval (hours)	Parenteral Dosage (gm/day)	Parenteral Interval (hours)	Usual Maximum Dose/day (gm)	Dosage Interval for Creatinine Clearance (ml/min) 80–50	50–10	Less than 10
Cephalexin	1–4	q6			4	6 hours	8–12 hours	24–48 hours
Cephradine	1–4	q6	2–8	q4–6	8	6 hours	8 hours	12–70 hours
Cefaclor	2	q6			2	(information not available)		
Cefadroxil	2	1 gm q12			2	12 hours	12 hours	24–36 hours
Cephalothin			2–12	q4–6	12	6 hours	8 hours	12 hours
Cefazolin			1–6	q6–8	6	12 hours	7/mg/kg q12h	5 mg/kg q24h
Cephaloridine[a]								
Cephapirin			2–6	q4–6	12			7.5–15 mg/kg q12h
Cefamandole			2–12	q4–6	12	6 hours	8 hours	12 hours
Cefoxitin			3–8	q6–8	8	8 hours	8–24 hours	12–48 hours

[a]Not recommended because of renal toxicity.

Table 3. Absorption and Biotransformation
of the Cephalosporins

Drug	Route of Administration	Protein Binding (%)
Cephalexin	Oral	10–15
Cephradine	Oral	10–15
Cefaclor	Oral	50
Cefadroxil	Oral	20
Cephalothin	Parenteral	60
Cefazolin	Parenteral	80
Cephaloridine	Parenteral	10–20
Cephapirin	Parenteral	50
Cefamandole	Parenteral	67–74
Cefoxitin	Parenteral	65–79

Note: All of these drugs are excreted by the kidney.

ABSORPTION AND BIOTRANSFORMATION

Table 3 gives information on the absorption and biotransformation
of the cephalosporins.

RECOMMENDED READING

Bernard, B., Barton, L., Abute, M., and Bullard, C.   Maternal-fetal transfer of
   cefazolin in the first twenty weeks of pregnancy. *J. Infect. Dis.* 136:377–
   382, 1977.
*Handbook of Antimicrobial Therapy. The Medical Letter on Drugs and
   Therapeutics* (Rev. ed.), New Rochelle, N.Y.: The Medical Letter, 1978.
Sanders, C. V., and Bourge, R. C.   When and how to use the new
   cephalosporins. *Contemp. Gynecol. Obstet.* 14:67–77, 1979.
Thompson, R. L.   The cephalosporins. *Mayo Clin. Proc.* 52:625, 1977.

(GRD)

Chloral Hydrate (Noctec®)

INDICATIONS AND RECOMMENDATIONS

The use of chloral hydrate during pregnancy is relatively contraindicated because other therapeutic agents are preferable. It has
sedative and hypnotic actions similar to those of paraldehyde, alcohol, and the barbiturates, and it is used primarily as a hypnotic
in the treatment of simple insomnia. Chloral hydrate and its active
metabolite, trichloroethanol, are known to cross the placental barrier rapidly after maternal administration. The effects of its use

during pregnancy have not been adequately studied. A British study of the pharmacokinetics of a single antepartum dose of chloral hydrate in 52 pregnant women and their offspring has been published. The authors report that no deleterious effects were noted in either mothers or neonates.

No sedative has been found to be absolutely safe during pregnancy, as most cross the placenta and produce sedation and withdrawal symptoms in the newborn. Should such therapy be required during pregnancy, phenobarbital may be used in the lowest dosage and frequency possible.

RECOMMENDED READING

Bernstine, J. B., Meyer, A. E., and Hayman, H. B.   Maternal and foetal blood estimation following the administration of chloral hydrate during labor. *J. Obstet. Gynaecol. Br. Emp.* 61:683–685, 1954.

Goodman, L. S., and Gilman, A.   *The Pharmacological Basis of Therapeutics* (5th ed.). New York: Macmillan, 1975. Pp. 127–129.

(EMT)

Chloramphenicol (Chloromycetin)

INDICATIONS AND RECOMMENDATIONS

Chloramphenicol should be avoided in late pregnancy and during labor because of the potential for the "gray syndrome" in the newborn infant. It should be used during pregnancy only for serious infections with organisms known to be sensitive to the drug. Because of the potential for life-threatening toxicity and hypersensitivity reactions, chloramphenicol should be used only when other antibiotics cannot be substituted. It may be necessary to use chloramphenicol to treat serious anaerobic infections, salmonella infections, and rickettsial diseases. It is also often used against *Hemophilus influenzae* meningitis and brain abscesses.

SPECIAL CONSIDERATIONS IN PREGNANCY

The "gray syndrome" may be seen in chloramphenicol-treated newborns, especially those born prematurely. The syndrome usually begins 2 to 9 days after therapy is begun. It consists of vomiting, refusal to suck, rapid irregular respiration and abdominal distension, followed in 24–48 hours by flaccidity, an ashen-gray color, and hypothermia. About 40% of these neonates die from circulatory collapse, usually on about the 5th day. It has been determined that newborns are unable to conjugate and excrete chloramphenicol, and the "gray syndrome" is related to toxic blood levels of the drug. Although toxic effects have not been observed in newborns whose mothers received as much as 1 gm of chloramphenicol every 2 hours during labor, it is probably best to avoid this drug just prior to delivery. Chloramphenicol does cross the placenta.

Because chloramphenicol appears in breast milk, it is best for nursing mothers not to use this drug.

DOSAGE

Chloramphenicol may be given orally, intramuscularly or intravenously. The usual oral dosage is 500 mg every 4 hours. The drug comes in capsules of 125 mg and 250 mg.

Intravenous dosage is the same as oral dosage, except for typhoid when a 2-gm loading dose is recommended.

Patients with renal disease should receive the usual dose of chloramphenicol, although anemia is more likely to occur. Patients with hepatic disease should receive reduced dosages and have serum levels monitored.

ADVERSE EFFECTS

Hypersensitivity Reactions. Chloramphenicol is the most common drug cause of pancytopenia. This effect is not dose-related, but is usually associated with prolonged oral therapy, especially with multiple exposures. The incidence is 1 in 40,000 courses of therapy. The longer the interval between the last dose of drug and the appearance of the first sign of blood dyscrasia, the greater the likelihood of fatality. When total aplasia of the bone marrow occurs, the fatality rate is almost 100%. Other hypersensitivity reactions include a macular or vesicular skin rash, hemorrhage from skin and mucous membranes, fever, and atrophic glossitis.

Toxic Effects. Anemia occurs in patients having plasma concentrations of chloramphenicol above 25 μg/ml. It is seen most often with parenteral therapy, is dose-related, and usually disappears completely about 12 days after discontinuance of therapy. The drug inhibits the uptake and incorporation of iron into heme, resulting in anemia, reticulocytopenia, and elevated plasma iron levels.

Chloramphenicol can also cause nausea, vomiting, diarrhea, and perineal irritation. The drug has a bitter taste when taken orally. This bitterness is also noted with rapid intravenous administration. Optic neuritis has been reported with chloramphenicol. Large oral doses may prolong the prothrombin time, presumably by altering the bacterial flora of the gastrointestinal tract.

Because of these relatively serious toxic and hypersensitivity effects, chloramphenicol should not be used for mild or self-limited infections, and should be considered contraindicated in pregnancy except in serious situations where other alternatives are not available.

MECHANISM OF ACTION

Chloramphenicol inhibits protein synthesis in bacteria and rickettsiae, primarily by preventing peptide bond synthesis in ribosomes.

ABSORPTION AND BIOTRANSFORMATION

Chloramphenicol is rapidly absorbed after oral ingestion, with significant plasma concentrations present at 30 minutes and peak levels attained in 2 hours. The half-life is 1½–3½ hours. Intramuscular administration gives lower plasma levels than intravenous or oral dosing, and it is probably most efficient to avoid this route, or to monitor serum levels if it is used.

The drug is inactivated in the liver by conjugation in a step mediated by glucuronyl transferase. The inactive metabolite is rapidly excreted in the urine. Over 80% of an oral dose can be recovered from the urine.

RECOMMENDED READING

Goodman, L. S., and Gilman, A. *The Pharmacological Basis of Therapeutics* (5th ed.). New York: Macmillan, 1975. Pp. 1194–1200.
Kucers, A., and Bennett, N. McK. *The Use of Antibiotics* (2nd ed.). London: William Heinemann, 1975. Pp. 244–270.

(DRC)

Chloroquine (Aralen®)

INDICATIONS AND RECOMMENDATIONS

The use of chloroquine during pregnancy should be limited to suppressive therapy in women entering areas with endemic malaria and to treatment of acute attacks of malaria. This drug should not be used for the treatment of inflammatory disease states in pregnancy.

SPECIAL CONSIDERATIONS IN PREGNANCY

When the drug was given in doses appropriate for malaria prophylaxis, 300–500 mg weekly, no studies have shown untoward fetal effects. Larger, anti-inflammatory doses taken during pregnancy, however, have resulted in spontaneous abortion and in vestibular and retinal damage in the fetus.

DOSAGE

When necessary for suppressive therapy of malaria, chloroquine phosphate 500 mg (300 mg of base) should be given weekly beginning 1 week prior to arrival, throughout the stay, and for 3 weeks after leaving the malarious area.

An initial loading dose of 1 gm is administered for treatment of an acute attack of vivax or falciparum malaria. This is followed by an additional 500 mg after 6–8 hours and 500 mg again on the 2 consecutive days. A total dose of 2.5 gm is given in 3 days. Anti-inflammatory doses range from 250–750 mg daily for prolonged periods.

ADVERSE EFFECTS

When used in antimalarial doses, side effects of chloroquine are mild and include transient headache, visual disturbances, gastrointestinal upset, and pruritis. Long-term therapy at anti-inflammatory doses may be associated with development of retinopathy, and irreversible visual loss may be sustained. Other side effects include dose-dependent myelosuppression, skin rashes, neuromyopathy, tinnitus and deafness, and electrocardiographic changes.

MECHANISM OF ACTION

The exact mechanisms of chloroquine's activity are unclear. Its antimalarial activity is thought to result from its binding to DNA and its selective accumulation in certain tissues, including parasitized erythrocytes. Chloroquine exerts no significant activity against exoerythrocytic stages of plasmodia.

Chloroquine rapidly controls the parasitemia and clinical symptoms of acute malarial attacks. Fever is controlled within 24–48 hours after administration of therapeutic doses. With the exception of certain strains, chloroquine completely cures falciparum malaria. Relapses of vivax malaria, however, are not prevented, although the intervals between relapses are substantially increased.

ABSORPTION AND BIOTRANSFORMATION

Chloroquine is rapidly and almost completely absorbed from the gastrointestinal tract. Much of the drug is bound to plasma proteins or to tissues; approximately 30% is metabolized. Chloroquine is cleared by the kidneys at a very slow rate, which may be increased by acidification of the urine. With single or weekly doses, the plasma half-life is approximately 3 days.

RECOMMENDED READING

Drugs for parasitic infections. *Med. Lett. Drugs Ther.* 20:20–21, 1978.

Dukes, N. M. G. (Ed.). *Myeler's Side Effects of Drugs, Vol. VIII.* New York: Excerpta Medica-American Elsevier, 1975.

Health Information for International Travel, 1978. *Morbid. Mortal. Weekly Rep.* 27:62–63, 1978.

Heinonen, O. P., Slone, D., and Shapiro, S. *Birth Defects and Drugs in Pregnancy.* Littleton, Mass.: Publishing Sciences Group, 1977. P. 299.

Pritchard, J. A., and MacDonald, P. C. (Eds.). *Williams Obstetrics* (15th ed.). New York: Appleton-Century-Crofts, 1976.

Shepard, T. H. *Catalog of Teratogenic Agents* (2nd ed.). Baltimore: Johns Hopkins University Press, 1976.

(TKH)

Chlorpheniramine (Chlor-Trimeton®)

INDICATIONS AND RECOMMENDATIONS

The use of chlorpheniramine during pregnancy should be limited to the provision of symptomatic relief of allergic symptoms caused by histamine release. These include urticaria, rhinitis, and pruritus. Because chlorpheniramine is an antihistamine that merely provides palliative therapy, the avoidance of allergens should be the primary treatment for these symptoms whenever possible. Chlorpheniramine does not appear to have teratogenic effects at recommended doses; however, no prospective studies are available. This drug is not recommended for use by lactating women.

SPECIAL CONSIDERATIONS IN PREGNANCY

No prospective studies that evaluate the safety of chlorpheniramine use during pregnancy have been conducted. One large retrospective study, however, found no evidence incriminating this drug as a teratogenic agent.

Due to its anticholinergic properties, chlorpheniramine may inhibit lactation. In addition, small amounts may be secreted into breast milk. This drug and all antihistamines, therefore, should be avoided by the lactating mother.

DOSAGE

The usual oral dose of chlorpheniramine is 2–4 mg three to four times a day. It is available in an extended-release formulation, 8–12 mg, that may be given twice to three times a day.

ADVERSE EFFECTS

Anticholinergic side effects are most common. These include dry mouth and eyes, and, rarely, blurred vision. Drowsiness, anorexia, nausea, epigastric distress, and dizziness may also be seen.

MECHANISM OF ACTION

Chlorpheniramine is a competitive antagonist of histamine that decreases edema formation by diminishing capillary dilatation and permeability. It has anticholinergic activity, produces drowsiness, and possesses local anesthetic activity when applied topically.

ABSORPTION AND BIOTRANSFORMATION

The drug is primarily metabolized in the liver, probably by hydroxylation followed by glucuronidation. Excretion is via the kidney.

RECOMMENDED READING

Goodman, L. S., and Gilman, A. *The Pharmacological Basis of Therapeutics* (5th ed.). New York: Macmillan, 1975. Pp. 608–609.

Greenberger, P., and Patterson, R. Safety of therapy for allergic symptoms during pregnancy. *Ann. Intern. Med.* 89:234–237, 1978.

Heinonen, O. P., Slone, D., and Shapiro, S. *Birth Defects and Drugs in Pregnancy*. Littleton, Mass.: Publishing Sciences Group, 1977. Pp. 322–334.

Nishimura, H., and Tanimura, T. *Aspects of the Teratogenicity of Drugs*. Amsterdam: Excerpta Medica, 1976.

(JRC)

Cholestyramine (Cuemid®, Questran®)

INDICATIONS AND RECOMMENDATIONS

Cholestyramine is safe to use for symptomatic relief of pruritus secondary to cholestasis of pregnancy. The patient's prothrombin time should be monitored and fat-soluble vitamins supplemented when this drug is administered.

SPECIAL CONSIDERATIONS IN PREGNANCY

Since cholestyramine is not absorbed, any problems associated with its administration would be related to fat-soluble vitamin deficiency or interactions with other drugs.

DOSAGE

Cholestyramine is given as 10–12 gm in an oral suspension in three divided (3–4 gm) doses before meals. Steatorrhea and malabsorption of fat-soluble vitamins do not occur with doses below 20–30 gm/day. Pruritus often recurs 1–2 days after withdrawal of the drug.

ADVERSE EFFECTS

Because cholestyramine is not absorbed from the gastrointestinal tract, most side effects are digestive. These include constipation, abdominal discomfort and distention, flatulence, nausea, vomiting, diarrhea, heartburn, anorexia, and steatorrhea. Deficiencies of fat-soluble vitamins (vitamins K, A) can occur. Cholestyramine also is described by most patients as having an unpleasant taste.

MECHANISM OF ACTION

Cholestyramine is a resin that combines with bile acids in the intestine to form an insoluble complex that is excreted in the feces. As a result, bile acids are partially removed from the enterohepatic circulation, which may reduce the systemic circulating bile acid concentration, thereby reducing skin levels of bile acids and decreasing pruritus.

RECOMMENDED READING

Burrow, G. N., and Ferris, T. F. (Eds.). *Medical Complications During Pregnancy*. Philadelphia: W. B. Saunders, 1975. P. 356.
Goodman, L. S., and Gilman, A. *The Pharmacological Basis of Therapeutics* (5th ed.). New York: Macmillan, 1975. P. 769.

(GRD)

Clindamycin (Cleocin®)

INDICATIONS AND RECOMMENDATIONS

The use of clindamycin during pregnancy should be limited to the treatment of infections suspected to be caused by *Bacteroides fragilis*. This drug has an antibacterial spectrum similar to that of lincomycin and erythromycin, although it is slightly more effective against sensitive bacteria. If diarrhea develops during the administration of this drug, proctoscopy should be performed. Therapy may be continued if proctoscopic findings are normal but should be stopped if pseudomembranous plaques are observed.

SPECIAL CONSIDERATIONS IN PREGNANCY

There are no unusual maternal effects during pregnancy. The drug rapidly crosses the placenta and is 90% bound to serum protein. Cord concentrations of the drug are approximately 50% of that found in the maternal circulation. There are no reports of adverse fetal reactions to clindamycin administration.

DOSAGE

The oral dose of clindamycin is 150–450 mg every 6 hours. The intramuscular or intravenous dose is 300–600 mg every 6 hours.

ADVERSE EFFECTS

Frequent side effects include diarrhea and allergic reactions. Pseudomembranous colitis has been reported in 2–10% of patients receiving clindamycin and is sometimes fatal. This condition can occur during treatment or 3–4 weeks after completion of therapy. It is not related to dose or to route of administration.

MECHANISM OF ACTION

Clindamycin inhibits protein synthesis by binding to bacterial ribosomes.

ABSORPTION AND BIOTRANSFORMATION

Clindamycin is nearly completely absorbed following oral administration. It may also be given parenterally. Most of the drug is metabolized in the liver to products excreted in the urine and bile. Only 10% of the drug is excreted unchanged in the urine. Little adjustment of dosage is required for patients in renal failure, but the dose must be decreased in patients with hepatic decompensation.

RECOMMENDED READING

Handbook of Antimicrobial Therapy. The Medical Letter on Drugs and Therapeutics (Rev. ed.). New Rochelle, N.Y.: The Medical Letter, 1978.
Tedesco, F. J. Clindamycin and colitis: A review. *J. Infect. Dis.* 135 (Suppl):595–598, 1977.
Weinstein, A. J., Gibbs, R. S., and Gallagher, M. Placental transfer of clin-

damycin and gentamicin in term pregnancy. *Am. J. Obstet. Gynecol.* 124:688–691, 1976.

(GRD)

Clomiphene Citrate (Clomid®)

INDICATIONS AND RECOMMENDATIONS

Clomiphene is contraindicated during pregnancy. There is no indication for its use during pregnancy since it is utilized to induce ovulation. Some women, however, not knowing that they are pregnant, may inadvertently continue to take clomiphene citrate during the first trimester.

Clomiphene works on the central nervous system at the hypothalamic level to block estrogen uptake. This results in increased follicle-stimulating hormone (FSH) production by the pituitary with a consequent increase in follicular estradiol production. The elevated estradiol level stimulates an LH surge during midcycle, which in turn causes ovulation to occur. Clomiphene is taken approximately 7–12 days prior to ovulation, and studies have shown most of it to be cleared at the time of conception.

Maternal side effects when this drug is taken during the first trimester include scotomata, nausea, and abdominal pain. Effects on the fetus are unknown. There is only one case reported in the literature of a congenital anomaly (cleft palate) that might have been related to clomiphene ingestion during pregnancy. A Swedish retrospective study of 159 pregnancies conceived after clomiphene therapy analyzed 141 births, including seven sets of twins. A slightly increased incidence of severe congenital malformations was found when this series was compared to data from the Swedish Register of Malformations and a detailed study from one of the two participating hospitals (5.4% vs. 3.2%). Although this might indicate a direct teratogenic effect of the drug, the authors of the study felt that it was more likely to be an expression of the subfertility that made clomiphene therapy necessary since the incidence of malformed infants was comparable to that in series reporting the results of gonadotropin therapy.

Clomiphene should not be administered during pregnancy. If it is inadvertently taken for a short course, however, the patient can be reassured that this drug will probably have no adverse effect on the fetus.

RECOMMENDED READING

Ahlgren, M., Kallen, B., and Rannevik, G. Outcome of pregnancy after clomiphene therapy. *Acta Obstet. Gynecol. Scand.* 55:371–375, 1976.

Asch, R. H., and Greenblatt, R. B. Update on the safety and efficacy of clomiphene citrate as a therapeutic agent. *J. Reprod. Med.* 17:175–180, 1976.

Huppert, L. C., and Wallach, E. C. Induction of ovulation with clomiphene citrate. *J. Reprod. Med.* 18:201–208, 1977.

(AHD)

Clonidine (Catapres®)

INDICATIONS AND RECOMMENDATIONS

Clonidine is relatively contraindicated during pregnancy because other therapeutic agents are preferable. It is an imidazoline derivative that can be used as an antihypertensive agent. Clonidine reduces blood pressure primarily by stimulating alpha adrenergic receptor sites in the hypothalamus and other vasomotor centers in the central nervous system. It also suppresses the release of renal renin.

Side effects include postural hypotension, fluid and sodium retention, drowsiness, and bowel disturbances. Occasionally a weakly positive Coombs test will result, and an acute hypertensive crisis may accompany abrupt withdrawal of the drug after prolonged therapy.

Despite one report of its successful use in 5 Australian obstetrical patients, the drug has been insufficiently evaluated to recommend its use during pregnancy. Other agents currently available can achieve the same objectives and have been more thoroughly studied.

RECOMMENDED READING

Frohlich, E. D. The sympathetic depressant anti-hypertensives. *Drug Ther.* 5:24–33, 1975.

Johnson, C. I., and Aickin, D. R. The control of high blood pressure during labour with clonidine (Catapres). *Med. J. Aust.* 2:132–135, 1971.

Kelly, J. V. Drugs used in the management of toxemia of pregnancy. *Clin. Obstet. Gynecol.* 20:395–410, 1977.

Martin, J. D. A critical survey of drugs used in the treatment of hypertensive crises of pregnancy. *Med. J. Aust.* 2:252–254, 1974.

Yudkin, J. S. Withdrawal of clonidine. *Lancet* 1:546, 1977.

(RLB)

Clotrimazole (Gyne-Lotrimin®, Lotrimin®)

INDICATIONS AND RECOMMENDATIONS

The use of clotrimazole during pregnancy should be limited to the topical treatment of vaginal and skin infections caused by susceptible yeast and fungi. These include *Candida albicans* and *Trichophyton* species. At this time there are no data implicating clotrimazole as a teratogen. This medication should not be applied vaginally when membranes have ruptured.

SPECIAL CONSIDERATIONS IN PREGNANCY

The use of clotrimazole for the treatment of vaginal candidiasis during pregnancy has been extensively studied. Although reports disagree as to the efficacy of clotrimazole with respect to other antifungal agents, none of the studies implicate the drug as a teratogen.

DOSAGE

For the treatment of vaginal candidiasis, 1 vaginal tablet or one applicator dose of the vaginal cream should be inserted high into the vagina for 7 consecutive nights.

ADVERSE EFFECTS

Untoward effects of clotrimazole therapy are uncommon and may include erythema, burning, stinging, edema, pruritus, urticaria, and general irritation of the skin or vagina.

MECHANISM OF ACTION

Clotrimazole is structurally unrelated to the other antifungal agents and appears to act by interfering with the phospholipid layer of the fungal membrane. It has broad-spectrum antifungal activity. Clotrimazole therapy is effective in the treatment of vulvovaginal candidiasis, tinea pedis, tinea cruris, tinea corporis, and tinea versicolor.

ABSORPTION AND BIOTRANSFORMATION

Clotrimazole has been found to be only slightly absorbed from skin and vaginal mucosa. Only 0.15% of the dose was recovered in the urine after it had been applied to inflamed skin. Serum levels of 0.05 μg/ml were achieved after administration of a single intravaginal 100 mg tablet.

RECOMMENDED READING

Frerich, W., and Gad, A.   The frequency of *Candida* infections in pregnancy and their treatment with clotrimazole. *Curr. Med. Res. Opin.* 4:640–644, 1977.

Goodman, L. S., and Gilman, A.   *The Pharmacological Basis of Therapeutics* (5th ed.). New York: Macmillan, 1975. P. 1242.

Haram, K., and Digranes, A.   Vulvovaginal candidiasis in pregnancy treated with clotrimazole. *Acta Obstet. Gynecol. Scand.* 57:453–455, 1978.

Svendsen, E.   Comparative evaluation of miconazole, clotrimazole and nystatin for the treatment of candidal vulvovaginitis. *Curr. Ther. Res.* 23:666–672, 1978.

Tan, C. G.   A comparative trial of six day therapy with clotrimazole and nystatin in pregnant patients with vaginal candidiasis. *Postgrad. Med.* 50(Suppl. 1): 102–105, 1974.

(EAC)

Colchicine

INDICATIONS AND RECOMMENDATIONS

Colchicine is contraindicated during pregnancy. It is used to relieve the pain of attacks of acute gouty arthritis and in the prophylactic treatment of recurrent gout attacks.

Colchicine reduces the inflammatory response to deposition of monosodium urate crystals in joint tissue in part by inhibiting polymorphonuclear leukocyte metabolism, mobility, and chemotaxis. It also inhibits cell division in metaphase by interfering with the mitotic spindle.

Colchicine is embryocidal in mice and rabbits. The risk of teratogenesis in humans is unknown. While receiving daily maintenance colchicine therapy for prevention of familial Mediterranean fever, five patients became pregnant and were followed through delivery. One of these women continued the drug throughout pregnancy and gave birth to a normal child. Of the four who stopped colchicine after pregnancy was detected, one had a spontaneous abortion in the second month and three gave birth to healthy infants.

There is concern that colchicine given during pregnancy will result in an increased frequency of Down's syndrome in the offspring by causing chromosomal nondisjunction. One study of lymphocyte cultures from three gouty patients on colchicine showed a significant increase in cells with abnormal numbers of chromosomes, both tetraploid and peridiploid, when compared to matched controls. In this report 2 out of 54 parents of 27 children with Down's syndrome were found to be on colchicine therapy.

Gout is uncommon in women and is rarely seen before menopause. If treatment of an acute attack becomes necessary, a short course of phenylbutazone may be required. An elevated serum uric acid is common in toxemia but rarely requires therapy. Probenecid has been safely used and is indicated for treatment of significant hyperuricemia in pregnancy.

For the couple planning to have a child, it is recommended that colchicine ingestion by *either* parent be discontinued 3 months prior to conception.

RECOMMENDED READING

American Hospital Formulatory Service. *Monograph for Colchicine.* Washington, D.C.: American Society of Hospital Pharmacists, 1973.

Burrow, G. N., and Ferris, T. F. (Eds.). *Medical Complications During Pregnancy.* New York: W.B. Saunders, 1975. P. 805.

Ferrcira, N. R., and Breoniconti. A. Trisomy after colchicine therapy (Letter). *Lancet* 2:1304, 1968.

Goodman, L. S., and Gilman, A. *The Pharmacological Basis of Therapeutics* (5th ed.). New York: Macmillan, 1975. Pp. 350–352.

Santhanogopalas, T. Serum uric acid levels and transaminase activities in toxemias of pregnancy. *J. Obstet. Gynecol. India* 15:561–567, 1965.

Zemer, D., Pras, M., Sohar, E., and Gafni, J. Colchicine in familial Mediterranean fever (Letter). *N. Engl. J. Med.* 294:170–171, 1976.

(CRV)

Contraceptives, Oral

INDICATIONS AND RECOMMENDATIONS

The use of oral contraceptives is contraindicated during pregnancy since there is no reason for their use. Some patients, however, not knowing that they have conceived, may inadvertently continue to take oral contraceptives early in the first trimester.

Combination oral contraceptive pills in the United States contain a 19 nortestosterone progestin and a synthetic estrogen. When taken during pregnancy these drugs may increase maternal nausea and vomiting and cause cholestatic jaundice. Important effects on the female fetus may include virilization of genital organs from the progestins, which act as weak androgens (e.g., clitoral hypertrophy and labial fusion). Extrapolating from diethylstilbestrol (DES) data the estrogens may cause vaginal adenosis and adenocarcinoma and in male fetuses, testicular cysts, oligospermia, and hypospadius. Progestins in the pill have also been associated with neural tube defects, limb and cardiac anomalies, and cleft palates when taken during the first trimester. The oral contraceptive steroids are secreted in the breast milk of nursing mothers.

The oral contraceptives are contraindicated in pregnancy because of potential adverse effects on the fetus. It goes without saying that they have no therapeutic value in pregnant women. Although an association has been noted between congenital anomalies and oral contraceptives taken during the first trimester, the risk of this occurring is probably small.

RECOMMENDED READING

Chez, R. A.   Proceedings of the symposium Progesterone, Progestins, and Fetal Development. *Fertil. Steril.* 30:16–26, 1978.

Heinonen, O. P., Slone, D., Monson, R. R., Hook, E. B., and Shapiro, S. Cardiovascular birth defects and antenatal exposure to female sex hormones. *N. Engl. J. Med.* 296:67–70, 1977.

Keith, L., and Berger, S. L.   The relationship between congenital defects and the use of exogenous progestational (contraceptive) hormones during pregnancy: A 20 year review. *Int. J. Gynecol. Obstet.* 15:115–124, 1977.

(AHD)

Corticosteroids: Dexamethasone (Decadron®), Hydrocortisone (Cortef®, Solu-Cortef®), Methylprednisolone (Medrol®, Solu-Medrol®), Prednisone (Deltasone®)

INDICATIONS AND RECOMMENDATIONS

Corticosteroid therapy may be administered during pregnancy and lactation if it is medically indicated. These agents are used as replacement therapy for acute or chronic adrenal insufficiency, as suppressive therapy for congenital adrenal hyperplasia, and in the treatment of a large number of pathological states as anti-inflammatory agents. They are also being increasingly used in obstetrics for the prevention of respiratory distress syndrome (RDS) in the neonate in situations in which premature delivery of the infant is likely.

When administered for maternal indications, it is recommended that prednisone be used in preference to other steroids whenever possible since it has the poorest transport across the placenta. Neonates should be observed for transient adrenocortical insufficiency when their mothers have received chronic steroid therapy during pregnancy.

Exogenous corticosteroid therapy to mothers with impending premature delivery remains a controversial subject. If steroids are to be used for this indication, the following guidelines should be followed:

1. They should not be given to patients who will be delivered of their infants less than 24 hours after initiation of therapy.
2. They should not be given after 34 weeks.
3. They should be used with caution in hypertensive patients until their effectiveness in this group of patients is better demonstrated.

SPECIAL CONSIDERATIONS IN PREGNANCY

Chronic maternal steroid ingestion during the first trimester has been associated with approximately a 1% incidence of cleft palate in human offspring. Because of animal studies suggesting an effect on neurological and pulmonary development in fetuses exposed to steroids in utero, caution is necessary in administering such drugs to pregnant women. Numerous reports document apparent normalcy in infants whose mothers had Cushing's syndrome or who were treated with steroids for other conditions throughout the pregnancy. Sporadic cases of transient adrenocortical insufficiency in such newborns have been reported. Well-controlled prospective studies have not been performed.

High-dose maternal glucocorticoid therapy has been shown to decrease the incidence of RDS in the offspring of women who are delivered of their infants prior to 34 weeks. Initial reports from investigators in New Zealand suggested that this relationship may not pertain when the mother is hypertensive, although subsequent studies have contested this point. Very little information exists about the long-term effects on infants whose mothers received bolus therapy in the third trimester. However, reports devoted to this question should start to appear soon; treatment of humans was begun in the early 1970s.

Large amounts of corticosteroids (75 mg cortisol per day) may suppress fetal adrenal production of estrogen precursor with subsequent lowering of plasma and urinary estriol values. In one series of 21 patients who received steroids during 29 pregnancies, however, there was no evidence of fetal adrenocortical insufficiency despite total doses of 11,000 mg of cortisone in one case and 6,250 mg of prednisone in another.

DOSAGE

The dosage of glucocorticoids varies depending upon the condition being treated. Table 4 lists the equivalent amounts for some of the available forms. For acute adrenal insufficiency the dosage of hydrocortisone is 100 mg IV every 8 hours, then 25 mg IM every 6–8 hours. The usual dose for the treatment of chronic adrenal insufficiency is 5–15 mg of hydrocortisone, or its equivalent, tid, guided by the patient's blood pressure and sense of well-being. Depending upon the form of steroid given and the patient's electrolyte picture, mineralocorticoids may need to be added.

For anteropituitary insufficiency, 25 mg of cortisone given upon arising and 12.5 mg in the late afternoon is adequate replacement and somewhat mimics the normal diurnal cycle. Higher-than-physiological doses are employed in the treatment of rheumatoid arthritis, systemic lupus erythematosus nephritis, autoimmune hemolytic anemia, renal transplantation, and other situations in which the immune response is to be depressed. For suppression of ce-

Table 4. Equivalent Amounts for Some Available Forms of Corticosteroids

Equivalent doses	Mg	Route of Administration
Cortisone	25	IM, PO
Hydrocortisone	20	IV, IM, PO
Prednisone	5	PO
Methylprednisolone	4	IV, IM, PO
Triamcinolone	4	IM, PO
Paramethasone	2	PO
Betamethasone	0.75	IV, IM, PO
Dexamethasone	0.75	IV, IM, PO

Data derived from G. W. Thorne, R. D. Adams, E. Braunwald, C. Isselbacher, and R. G. Petersdorf (Eds.). *Harrison's Principles of Internal Medicine* (8th ed.). New York: McGraw-Hill, 1977. P. 554.

rebral edema, the conventional dosage is 100 mg prednisone per day in divided doses (equivalent to 400 mg hydrocortisone).

Asthmatics requiring steroid therapy for an acute attack are generally started at 100 mg cortisol (Solu-Cortef®) IV every 8 hours, then placed on oral prednisone 20–40 mg every day, after which the dose is tapered rapidly. Steroids are used in retention enemas for refractory ulcerative colitis, as eye drops for nonbacterial and nonviral inflammatory conditions, and as creams and lotions for various dermatological conditions. These topical forms are systemically absorbed, especially through inflamed hyperemic tissues.

In an ongoing collaborative NIH-sponsored study, the dose of dexamethasone administered for the antenatal prevention of RDS is 5 mg IM every 6 hours × 4. In earlier studies a mixture of betamethasone phosphate and acetate at a dose of 12 mg IM every 24 hours × 2 was utilized.

ADVERSE EFFECTS

Side effects include fluid and electrolyte imbalance, hyperglycemia, peptic ulcers (that may bleed or perforate), susceptibility to infections (including tuberculosis), osteoporosis, psychosis, myopathy, striae, ecchymoses, acne, and fat deposition characteristic of Cushing's syndrome.

MECHANISM OF ACTION

Corticosteroids are a family of 21-carbon compounds. Their action is dependent upon specific cytoplasmic receptors that, when combined with the steroid, migrate to the cell nucleus, after which enzyme synthesis is influenced. Their physiological effects are widespread. They stabilize lysosomal membranes, inhibiting the production and release of inflammatory mediators and decreasing chemotaxis. They also decrease mast cell activity and lymphocyte lysis, which consequently disturbs cell-mediated immunity.

Hematological effects include granulocytosis (due to demargination of white blood cells), increased platelets, and decreased eosinophils.

Metabolic effects include increased peripheral gluconeogenesis, hepatic glycogenolysis, and hepatic gluconeogenesis. In the presence of growth hormone, corticosteroids promote lipolysis. Electrolyte changes include sodium and water retention, along with potassium loss in the urine.

Table 5. Anti-inflammatory and Sodium-retaining Potencies of Various Corticosteroid Compounds

Compound	Relative Anti-inflammatory Potency	Relative Sodium-retaining Potency
Hydrocortisone (cortisol)	1	1
Tetrahydrocortisol	0	0
Prednisone (Δ^1-cortisone)	4	0.8
Prednisolone (Δ^1-cortisol)	4	0.8
6α-methylprednisolone	5	0.5
9α-fluorocortisol	10	125
11-desoxycortisol	0	0
Cortisone	0.8	0.8
Corticosterone	0.35	15
11-desoxycorticosterone	0	100
Aldosterone	?	3000
Triamcinolone (9α-fluoro-16α-hydroxyprednisolone)	5	0
Paramethasone (6α-fluoro-16α-methylprednisolone)	10	0
Betamethasone (9α-fluoro-16β-methylprednisolone)	25	0
Dexamethasone (9α-fluoro-16α-methylprednisolone)	25	0

Adapted from L. S. Goodman, and A. Gilman. *The Pharmacological Basis of Therapeutics* (5th ed.). New York: Macmillan, 1975. Pp. 1480, 1491.

ABSORPTION AND BIOTRANSFORMATION

Some of the available corticosteroid compounds are well absorbed orally while others must be given parenterally (see Table 4). All biologically active adrenocortical steroids and their synthetic congeners have a double bond in the 4–5 position. Reduction of this bond can occur at hepatic or extrahepatic sites to yield an inactive compound. Conversion occurs, primarily in the liver, to sulfate esters or glucuronides; excretion is then via the kidneys.

RECOMMENDED READING

Baden, M., Bauer, C. R., Colle, E., Klein, G., Taeusch, H. W., and Stern, L. A controlled trial of hydrocortisone therapy in infants with respiratory distress syndrome. *Pediatrics* 50:526–534, 1972.

Challis, J. R., Kendall, J. Z., and Robinson, J. S. The regulation of corticosteroids during late pregnancy and their role in parturition. *Biol. Reprod.* 16:57–69, 1977.

Goodman, L. S., and Gilman, A. *The Pharmacological Basis of Therapeutics* (5th ed.). New York: Macmillan, 1975. Pp. 1477–1502.

Liggins, G. C., and Howie, R. N. A controlled trial of antepartum glucocorticoid treatment for prevention of the respiratory distress syndrome in premature infants. *Pediatrics* 50:515–525, 1972.

Murphy, B. E. P., Patrick, J., and Denton, R. L. Cortisol in amniotic fluid during human gestation. *J. Clin. Endocrinol. Metab.* 40:164–167, 1975.

Schapiro, S. Some physiologic biochemical and behavioral consequences of neonatal hormone administration: Cortisol and thyroxin. *Gen. Comp. Endocrinol.* 10:214–228, 1968.

Thorne, G. W., Adams, R. D., Braunwald, E., Isselbacher, C., Petersdorf, R. G. (Eds.). *Harrison's Principles of Internal Medicine* (8th ed.). New York: McGraw-Hill, 1977. P. 554.

Update: Drugs in Breast Milk. *Med. Lett. Drugs Ther.* 21:21, 1979.

Yackel, D. B., Kempers, R. D., and McConahey, W. M. Adrenocorticosteroid therapy in pregnancy. *Am. J. Obstet. Gynecol.* 96:985–989, 1966.

(BRS)

Coumarin Anticoagulants: Warfarin (Coumadin®, Panwarfin®)

INDICATIONS AND RECOMMENDATIONS

The use of oral anticoagulants in the warfarin family is contraindicated during the first trimester, because of their potential for causing severe fetal anomalies, and late in the third trimester, because of the associated deaths from fetal hemorrhage occurring during labor. Their use during the intervening period is controversial.

Long-term anticoagulation is indicated in the treatment of deep venous thromboembolic disease, prevention of clotting in arterial and cardiac surgery, and the prevention of clotting when prosthetic devices such as heart valves have been implanted. Some authors have advocated the use of the warfarin anticoagulants during the second trimester and up to three weeks prior to the delivery date in the third trimester. This approach, however, presupposes that premature labor and delivery will not occur, and this obviously can never be predicted with assurance. Anticoagulation of a premature infant during labor may be particularly disastrous because such infants are more susceptible to death from intracranial hemorrhage than full-term infants *without* this added complication. Furthermore, the cases of death in utero occurring during midpregnancy cause concern about the use of these agents even when their administration is confined to the second trimester. We therefore recommend that heparin be used throughout the pregnancy, despite the acknowledged risk of maternal osteoporosis associated with the administration of this agent for periods of more than 6 months.

Although warfarin passes into the breast milk of nursing mothers, it has not been associated with bleeding problems in their infants. Caution nevertheless should be advised in this situation, and periodic clotting studies should be performed in nursing infants whose mothers are taking oral anticoagulants.

SPECIAL CONSIDERATIONS IN PREGNANCY

No unusual maternal effects have been reported. Warfarin therapy, however, has been associated with severe fetal malformations when it has been taken during the first trimester. These include nasal hypoplasia, stippling of bone, ophthalmological abnormalities, intrauterine growth retardation, and developmental delay. In addition to the possible teratogenic effect of these compounds, they readily cross the placental barrier and anticoagulate the fetus. This has been associated with fetal hemorrhage, particularly when the mother is taking the drug around the time of delivery. There have also been isolated reports of fetal hemorrhage occurring in the second and third trimesters prior to labor, resulting in the birth of stillborn infants.

Warfarin passes into breast milk but has not been reported to cause hemorrhage in nursing infants.

DOSAGE

Warfarin (Coumadin®, Panwarfin®) is available in a number of different dosage strength tablets. Coumadin® is also available in an injectable form, although it is rarely used. Many authorities feel that a loading dose should be avoided; they advocate initiating therapy with 10 mg daily and then following the patient closely by laboratory monitoring. An alternative approach is to administer a loading dose of 20 mg followed by 10 mg in 24 hours. The amount of subsequent doses would depend on laboratory tests.

Warfarin therapy should be monitored by following the prothrombin time (PT), which should be maintained at one and one-half to two times control values. Heparin also prolongs this lab test; therefore, when using combined therapy while switching from heparin to a coumarin derivative, blood sampling should be done immediately prior to the scheduled heparin dose.

ADVERSE EFFECTS

The major maternal toxic effect of the drug is hemorrhage. Excessive bleeding may require the administration of fresh frozen plasma. Overdosage may be managed by giving vitamin K intravenously or subcutaneously. Less frequently encountered side effects include alopecia, dermatitis, nausea, vomiting, diarrhea, and a hypersensitivity reaction consisting of hemorrhagic infarction and necrosis of skin.

The following drugs given concurrently will diminish the response to oral anticoagulants: griseofulvin, barbiturates, glutethimide, vitamin K, and possibly estrogens and adrenocorticosteroids. Drugs that may enhance the response to the oral anticoagulants include: broad-spectrum antibiotics, salicylates, anabolic steroids, chloramphenicol, chloral hydrate, and phenylbutazone.

MECHANISM OF ACTION

Although there are many oral anticoagulants available for clinical use, the intermediate-acting preparations such as warfarin (Coumadin® and Panwarfin®) in the United States and phenprocoumon (Marcouran®) in Europe are used almost exclusively. Dicumerol® is no longer widely used because of its relatively poor gastrointestinal absorption.

Oral anticoagulants block the hepatic synthesis of factors II, VII, IX, and X by competitively inhibiting the action of vitamin K. Warfarin compounds may also directly affect the transportation of vitamin K to its site of action. An increased level of antithrombin III found in the plasma of patients taking oral anticoagulants may increase the antithrombotic effect.

By inhibiting the vitamin K–dependent factors, both the intrinsic and extrinsic coagulation cascades are altered. Warfarins have no direct effect on clotting factors that are already circulating. The anticoagulant effect is initiated as the coagulation factors disappear from the blood in proportion to their rates of degradation. The half-life of VII is 5 hours; of IX and X, 20–30 hours; of II, 100 hours.

ABSORPTION AND BIOTRANSFORMATION

Warfarin is readily and almost completely absorbed after oral administration. Ninety-seven percent of the drug is weakly bound to albumin in plasma. It accumulates in lung, liver, spleen, and kidney. The half-life in man is 15–55 hours. The lag time between peak plasma concentration and therapeutic response is a manifestation of the time required for depletion of circulating clotting factors and for the establishment of a plateau concentration. Warfarin is metabolized in the liver and metabolites of the drug are excreted in the urine. Some unabsorbed drug may pass into the feces. Warfarin anticoagulants pass the placental barrier and are excreted in the breast milk of nursing mothers.

RECOMMENDED READING

Hirsh, J., Cade, J. F., and O'Sullivan, E. F. Clinical experience with anticoagulant therapy during pregnancy. *Br. Med. J.* 1:270–273, 1970.

Koch-Weser, J., and Sellers, E. M. Drug interactions with coumarin anticoagulants. *N. Engl. J. Med.* 285:487–498, 1971.

O'Reilly, R. A., and Aggeler, P. M. Studies of coumarin anticoagulant drugs. Initiation of warfarin therapy without a loading dose. *Circulation* 38:169–173, 1968.

Shaul, W. L., Emery, H., and Hall, J. G. Chondroplasia puncta and maternal warfarin use during pregnancy. *Am. J. Dis. Child.* 129:360–362, 1975.

Tejani, N. Anticoagulant therapy with cardiac valve prostheses during pregnancy. *Obstet. Gynecol.* 42:785–793, 1973.

Villasanta, U. Thromboembolic disease in pregnancy. *Am. J. Obstet. Gynecol.* 93:142–160, 1965.

(MCM)

Cromolyn Sodium (Aarane®, Intal®)

INDICATIONS AND RECOMMENDATIONS

Cromolyn sodium may be administered to pregnant asthmatics prior to unavoidable exposure to allergens that have been proved to cause severe bronchospasm and to prevent exercise-induced bronchospasm. This drug seems to be well tolerated in pregnancy, and its systemic absorption is minimal. Cromolyn sodium has no role in the treatment of acute asthmatic attacks.

SPECIAL CONSIDERATIONS IN PREGNANCY

No unusual maternal effects are reported. No information is available regarding the passage of cromolyn sodium across the placenta.

Teratogenicity has not been reported in humans. Studies in animals have failed to produce teratogenesis after prolonged intravenous administration of the drug. Decreased fetal weight, however, has been reported in association with doses close to those that produce maternal toxicity in animals.

DOSAGE

The usual dose is 20 mg inhaled every 6 hours prn. A clinical response to this drug is often seen within 3 to 5 days but may take as long as a month.

Cromolyn sodium is only effective in exercise-induced bronchospasm if taken 1–20 minutes prior to the exercise. This drug should not be given during an acute asthmatic attack because it can aggravate the existing bronchial irritation.

ADVERSE EFFECTS

Side effects include mild sore throat, nasal congestion, cough, transient wheezing, urticaria, and maculopapular rash. Occasionally, angioedema, fever, nausea, vomiting, pulmonary infiltrates, muscular weakness, pericarditis, and anaphylaxis may occur.

MECHANISM OF ACTION

Cromolyn sodium inhibits the release of histamine and slow-reacting substance of anaphylaxis by mast cells. These are the chemical mediators of a bronchospastic response following either immunological or nonimmunological stimulation. This drug does not have direct bronchodilator, antihistaminic, or anti-inflammatory effects. The amount of drug absorbed into the circulation following inhalation of therapeutic doses does not appear to exert any generalized pharmacological action.

ABSORPTION AND BIOTRANSFORMATION

The drug is marketed as a crystallized powder, with lactose as an inert propellant, in a gelatin capsule. It is administered via a special inhaler. Only 1 to 2 mg of the 20-mg dose reaches the alveoli. The remainder is retained in the trachea and oropharynx and is swallowed later. Eight percent of the drug is absorbed systemically in the lung and gastrointestinal tract. Eighty percent of the cromolyn sodium is eliminated in the feces. The absorbed drug is excreted unchanged in the urine. The plasma half-life is 60–90 minutes.

RECOMMENDED READING

Berstein, I. L., Siegel, S. C., Brandon, M. L., Brown, E. B., Evans, R. R., Feinberg, A. R., Friedlander, S., Krumholz, R. A., Hadley, R. A., Handelman, N. I., Thurston, D., and Yamahe, M.   A controlled study of cromolyn sodium sponsored by the Drug Committee of the American Academy of Allergy. *J. Allergy Clin. Immunol.* 50:235–245, 1972.

Block, S. H.   Nasal congestion as a side effect of cromolyn sodium. *J. Allergy Clin. Immunol.* 53:243–244, 1974.

Falliers, C. J.   Cromolyn sodium (Editorial). *J. Allergy* 47:298, 1971.

Falliers, C. J.   Cromolyn sodium prophylaxis. *Pediatr. Clin. North Am.* 22:141–146, 1975.

Gwin, E., Kerby, G., and Ruth, W.   Cromolyn sodium in the treatment of asthma associated with aspirin hypersensitivity and nasal polyps. *Chest* 72:148–153, 1977.

Khurana, S., and Hyde, J. S.   Cromolyn sodium, five to six years later. *Ann. Allergy* 39:94–98, 1977.

Sheffer, A., Rocklin, R., and Goetzl, E.   Immunologic components of hypersensitivity reactions to cromolyn sodium. *N. Engl. J. Med.* 293:1220–1224, 1975.

Silverman, M., and Andrea, T.   Time course of effect of disodium cromoglycate on exercise-induced asthma. *Arch. Dis. Child.* 47:419–422, 1972.

(RJR)

Cyclizine (Marezine®)

INDICATIONS AND RECOMMENDATIONS

Cyclizine is safe to use during pregnancy for the prevention of nausea, vomiting, and dizziness associated with motion sickness. This drug is probably effective for control of postoperative nausea and vomiting when used parenterally or rectally. Although cyclizine has been shown to be teratogenic in rodents, this effect has not been demonstrated in humans when recommended doses are used.

SPECIAL CONSIDERATIONS IN PREGNANCY

Cyclizine crosses the placenta and has been shown to be teratogenic in rodents. However, large-scale studies in humans show that the rate of severe congenital anomalies in children of mothers who took cyclizine during pregnancy is not significantly different than in the offspring of mothers who did not receive antinauseants.

DOSAGE

The dose for prevention of motion sickness is 50 mg ½ hr prior to departure, repeating every 4–6 hours prn. Dose should not exceed 200 mg/day.

For prevention of postoperative vomiting the dose is 50 mg IM every 4–6 hours or 100 mg rectally ever 4–6 hours.

ADVERSE EFFECTS

The more common side effects of cyclizine include drowsiness, dry mouth, and, rarely, blurred vision.

MECHANISM OF ACTION

Cyclizine is a piperazine antihistamine that depresses labyrinth excitability and vestibular-cerebellar pathway conduction. It inhibits the effects of histamine on capillary permeability and on smooth muscle by competitive inhibition at H_1 receptors. Either stimulation or depression of the central nervous system may occur through an unknown mechanism. It has anticholinergic activity, although no significant effects on the cardiovascular system occur at normal therapeutic doses.

ABSORPTION AND BIOTRANSFORMATION

Cyclizine is readily absorbed from the gastrointestinal tract and is widely distributed to body tissues. The exact nature of elimination in humans is unknown, but it appears to be extensively metabolized in the liver and excreted in the urine.

RECOMMENDED READING

Biggs, J. S. G.   Vomiting in pregnancy: Causes and management. *Drugs* 9:299–306, 1975.

Goodman, L. S., and Gilman, A.   *The Pharmacological Basis of Therapeutics* (5th ed.). New York: Macmillan 1975. Pp. 608–611.

Heinonen, D., Slone, D., and Shapiro, S.   *Birth Defects and Drugs in Pregnancy*. Littleton, Mass.: Publishing Sciences Group, 1977. Pp. 323–333.

Long, J. W.   *The Essential Guide to Prescription Drugs* (1st ed.). New York: Harper & Row, 1977. Pp. 206–208.

Milkovich, L., and Van den Berg, B. J.   An evaluation of the teratogenicity of certain antinauseant drugs. *Am. J. Obstet. Gynecol.* 125:244–248, 1976.

Nishimura, H., and Tanimura, T.   *Clinical Aspects of the Teratogenicity of Drugs*. Amsterdam: Excerpta Medica, 1976.

(DJK)

Dextran: Dextran 70 (Macrodex®), Dextran 40 (Rheomacrodex®)

INDICATIONS AND RECOMMENDATIONS

Dextran is relatively contraindicated during pregnancy because other therapeutic agents, for example, heparin, are preferable. This compound has been used in thromboembolism prophylaxis and as a plasma expander.

The antithrombotic actions of dextran include reduced platelet adhesiveness, platelet factor III depression, altered fibrin clot structure, and hemodilution of clotting factors. Factors V, VII, IX, and fibrinogen are decreased more than might be expected by hemodilution.

Dextran is available in a high molecular weight (MW) form (MW 70,000, Macrodex®) and a low molecular weight form (MW 40,000, Rheomacrodex®). Most of the former is sequestered by the reticuloendothelial system and slowly metabolized over days to weeks. The latter is readily filtered by the kidney with little reabsorption. While most authors have not found significant differences in the effectiveness of the two forms, some have reported better results with the Dextran 70. This may be due to its prolonged clearance or a failure to infuse Dextran 40 for a sufficiently long period.

Adverse effects include severe anaphylactic reactions as well as minor allergic responses such as rash, urticaria, nausea, and vomiting. Some bacterial polysaccharides demonstrate cross-sensitivity to dextrans. These include Group H streptococci, pneumococci, and types II, XII, and XX *Salmonella typhosa*. Plasma expansion may precipitate congestive heart failure in a borderline compensated cardiac patient. Finally, the following laboratory tests may be artificially altered: blood glucose, bilirubin, total serum protein, and cross matches.

No information is available regarding adverse fetal effects.

Dextran is an effective plasma expander, and it reduces the incidence of thromboembolic disease when administered prophylactically. However, in patients with hypovolemia secondary to blood loss, clotting problems may be aggravated; in patients with infection caused by streptococci, pneumococci, and *Salmonella*, the risk of anaphylaxis may increase. There may also be interference created with blood cross-matching at a time when this is critical. It is therefore recommended that heparin be used for the prophylaxis and therapy of thromboembolic disorders during pregnancy and that more physiological plasma expanders be used preferentially.

RECOMMENDED READING

Atik, M. Dextran 40 and dextran 70, a review. *Arch. Surg.* 94:664–672, 1967.

Data, J. L., and Nies, A. S. Dextran 40. *Ann. Intern. Med.* 81:500–504, 1974.

(MCM)

Dextromethorphan (over-the-counter)

INDICATIONS AND RECOMMENDATIONS

Dextromethorphan is safe to use during pregnancy. It is used for its antitussive properties.

SPECIAL CONSIDERATIONS IN PREGNANCY

Respiratory depression in the fetus is a theoretical possibility if a pregnant woman with severely impaired renal function takes the drug chronically up to the time of delivery.

DOSAGE

The usual dose is 10 to 20 mg three or four times a day. It is generally administered in syrup form, with 5 cc containing 10–15 mg of dextromethorphan. It is also available as a lozenge. An effect is usually observed within 30 minutes.

ADVERSE EFFECTS

Unlike codeine, dextromethorphan rarely produces drowsiness or gastrointestinal disturbances. Its toxicity is low, but in very high doses it may produce central nervous system depression.

MECHANISM OF ACTION

Dextromethorphan is the *d*-isomer of the codeine analog of levorphanol, but it has no analgesic or addictive properties. The drug acts centrally, raising the threshold for coughing.

ABSORPTION AND BIOTRANSFORMATION

Metabolism is believed to occur in the liver with excretion in the kidney.

RECOMMENDED READING

Goodman, L. S., and Gilman, A. *The Pharmacological Basis of Therapeutics* (5th ed.). New York: Macmillan, 1975. P. 279.

Nelson, M. M., and Forfar, J. O. Association between drugs administered during pregnancy and congenital abnormalities of the fetus. *Br. Med. J.* 1:523–527, 1971.

Schenkel, B., and Vorherr, H. Non-prescription drugs during pregnancy: Potential teratogenic and toxic effects upon embryo and fetus. *J. Reprod. Med.* 12:27–45, 1974.

(RAC)

Diazepam (Valium®)

INDICATIONS AND RECOMMENDATIONS

The use of diazepam during pregnancy should be limited to the control of status epilepticus and the intermittent treatment of anxiety states. This drug is widely used in the nonpregnant patient as a sedative, during hallucinogenic "bad trips," and in the management of opiate or alcohol withdrawal. It is the drug of choice for the treatment of status epilepticus but is not useful in the chronic management of epilepsy. Diazepam has been used to control eclamptic seizures, although magnesium sulfate is the drug of choice prior to delivery. Chronic use of diazepam during pregnancy is associated with significant adverse effects in the neonate and is therefore not recommended.

As diazepam is excreted into breast milk and may cause lethargy, weight loss, and sedation in the nursing infant, its use by the lactating mother is not recommended.

SPECIAL CONSIDERATIONS IN PREGNANCY

Diazepam rapidly crosses the placental barrier with fetal-maternal equilibrium being reached within 1 hour in humans. Benzodiazepine concentrations in cord blood or fetal plasma have been reported to exceed the levels in maternal blood. This may be due to their marked lipid solubility and delayed metabolism by the immature fetal liver.

Loss of beat-to-beat fetal heart rate variability has been reported within 2 minutes of the intravenous administration of 20 mg of diazepam. This effect lasts approximately 60 minutes and does not affect fetal pH or Apgar score. Loss of long-term variability has also been noted.

Use of diazepam has been associated with cleft lip in the neonate but has not been proved to be causative. Neonatal diazepam withdrawal symptoms have been reported following second and third trimester maternal ingestion of 15–20 mg of diazepam per day for at least 12 weeks. The symptoms were similar to neonatal narcotic withdrawal symptoms. Severe neonatal respiratory depression can occur when diazepam is used in high doses for control of eclampsia.

Diazepam administered parenterally to the mother has been shown to cause an elevation of neonatal serum bilirubin concentrations secondary to delayed bilirubin metabolism. This effect is dose-dependent. In addition, injectable diazepam contains sodium benzoate, a buffer known to displace bilirubin from albumin in vitro.

Diazepam and its metabolite, N-demethyldiazepam, are excreted into human breast milk. It has been implicated as a cause of lethargy, sedation, and weight loss in the nursing infant.

DOSAGE

The usual dosage range for chronic oral therapy is from 2 mg at bedtime for the treatment of mild anxiety associated with insomnia to as much as 20 mg tid for management of alcohol withdrawal, severe anxiety, or muscle spasm. Doses of 30 mg given intravenously may be required to control status epilepticus.

ADVERSE EFFECTS

Side effects most commonly encountered are drowsiness, ataxia, and lethargy. Paradoxical effects such as increased hostility or anxiety have been reported. Excessive intravenous administration or intravenous therapy in the presence of other central nervous system depressants can produce significant respiratory depression. Chronic administration can lead to drug dependence.

MECHANISM OF ACTION

The exact mechanism of action of diazepam is still under investigation. This drug suppresses the spread of seizure activity produced by epileptogenic foci. Its effects are thought to be mediated in the central nervous system, perhaps by mimicking the effects of the inhibitory neurotransmitter, glycine.

ABSORPTION AND BIOTRANSFORMATION

Diazepam is rapidly absorbed from the gastrointestinal tract and becomes highly protein-bound in plasma. It is metabolized in the liver to hydroxylated derivatives and to N-demethyldiazepam, an active metabolite. After saturation of tissue stores, the half-life of diazepam is 24–48 hours. Following glucuronic acid conjugation, the metabolites are excreted in the urine.

RECOMMENDED READING

Cole, A. P., and Hailey, D. M.   Diazepam and active metabolites in breast milk and their transfer to the neonate. *Arch. Dis. Child. 50:741*–742, 1975.

Eadie, M. J., and Tyrer, J. H. *Anticonvulsant Therapy.* Edinburgh: Churchill-Livingstone, 1974.

Erkkola, R., and Kanto, J.   Diazepam and breast feeding. *Lancet* 1:1235–1236, 1972.

Erkkola, R., Kangas, L., and Pekkarinen, A.   The transfer of diazepam across the placenta during labor. *Acta Obstet. Gynecol. Scand.* 52:165–170, 1973.

Goodman, L. S., and Gilman, A.   *The Pharmacological Basis of Therapeutics* (5th ed.). New York: Macmillan, 1975. Pp. 189–192.

Mofid, M., Brinkman, C. R., and Assali, N. S.   Effects of diazepam on utero-placental and fetal hemodynamic metabolism. *Obstet. Gynecol.* 41: 364–368, 1973

Patrick, M. J., Tilstone, W. J., and Reavey, P.   Diazepam and breast feeding. *Lancet* 1:542–543, 1972.

Woodbury, D. M., Penry, J. K., and Schmidt, R. P.   *Antiepileptic Drugs.* New York: Raven Press, 1972.

(PHR)

Diazoxide (Hyperstat®)

INDICATIONS AND RECOMMENDATIONS

The use of diazoxide during pregnancy is controversial and if used at all should be reserved for patients with *severe* acute hypertensive episodes. This drug is a potent and rapidly acting antihypertensive agent and is marketed for the intravenous therapy of hypertensive emergencies. An oral preparation is available for the treatment of hypoglycemia, but this should not be used during pregnancy.

Diazoxide is rarely the drug of choice for the treatment of hypertension during pregnancy. When it is administered, the patient should have an intravenous infusion running and ideally should have been given sufficient fluid therapy prior to its use so as to raise the central venous pressure to measurable levels. The fetal heart rate should concurrently be monitored electronically. The mother's blood sugars should be monitored regularly and a cord blood glucose obtained from the neonate immediately after delivery. Whenever possible this drug should not be used in combination with either hydralazine or methyldopa.

Hypotensive episodes following diazoxide administration should be treated with the rapid infusion of 1 or more liters of 5% dextrose in normal saline. The use of sympathomimetic agents such as norepinephrine to restore the blood pressure should be avoided unless there is no response to the infusion of fluid. This should almost never be necessary.

SPECIAL CONSIDERATIONS IN PREGNANCY

The most serious potential side effect after the intravenous administration of a bolus of diazoxide to a toxemic patient is significant hypotension. Several series have shown some diastolic pressure drops to 50–60 mm Hg in patients with initial readings of 110 mm Hg or higher. In a number of these patients there was also concomitant fetal bradycardia. Severe hypotensive responses have been specifically related to the potentiating effects of other vasodilators (e.g., hydralazine) or catecholamine-depleting drugs (e.g., methyldopa or reserpine) given either prior to or subsequent to the administration of diazoxide.

Because sodium and water are retained when diazoxide is used, the concomitant use of furosemide has been advised for the medical patient. The use of potent diuretics, however, is probably ill-advised in toxemic patients with significant hypovolemia.

Since diazoxide stops uterine contractions and termination of the pregnancy is an integral part of the management of severely hypertensive, toxemic patients, intravenous oxytocin to induce labor must be given if vaginal delivery is to be accomplished. Hyperglycemia must be looked for in both mother and neonate.

Diazoxide crosses the placenta, but when it is given intravenously it seems to have little effect on the fetus. Some fetal hyperglycemia may be produced, but there are very few circulatory alterations. The fetus seems to rapidly metabolize the drug.

When diazoxide is given orally to pregnant women for several weeks, newborn alopecia, hypertrichosis lanuginosa, and decreased bone age have been reported.

DOSAGE

The usual intravenous dose is 300 mg or 5 mg/kg body weight. Maximum effectiveness is achieved by rapidly injecting the full dose of the drug within 10–30 seconds. The dependence of the hypotensive effect on the injection rate is related to the rapidity with which the drug is bound by serum albumin. The hypotensive effect will be noted within 5 minutes; thereafter, blood pressure increases gradually and returns to pretreatment levels within 3–15 hours. If the initial response is unsatisfactory, the dose may be repeated in 30 minutes.

ADVERSE EFFECTS

Since cardiovascular reflexes and the sympathetic nervous system function normally, diazoxide rarely causes postural hypotension. Sodium and water retention usually occur because of the drug's direct tubular antinatriuretic effect. Hyperglycemia may occur because of reduced insulin secretion by the pancreatic beta cells as well as a direct effect on the liver to increase its rate of glucose release. Mild hyperuricemia may be noted. A direct relaxation of uterine musculature can cause labor to stop. Finally, symptoms associated with the sympathetic reflex response to vasodilatation may occur.

MECHANISM OF ACTION

Diazoxide relaxes smooth muscle in all circulatory beds, which results in a reduction of vascular resistance. In association with this reduction in arterial pressure, there is a reflex increase in heart rate, stroke volume, and cardiac output, which may partially counteract the hypotensive effect of the vascular dilatation. Blood flow through all circulatory beds is generally well maintained and renal blood flow and glomerular filtration rate are usually unchanged or increased.

ABSORPTION AND BIOTRANSFORMATION

The drug is primarily eliminated from the body by glomerular filtration. The serum half-life is normally 20–30 hours, but 90% of the drug is rapidly bound to albumin after intravenous administration. Since only the free drug is active, diazoxide must be administered every 4–12 hours, despite the long half-life in serum.

RECOMMENDED READING

Henrich, W. L., Cronin, R., Miller, P. D., and Anderson, R. J.   Hypotensive sequelae of diazoxide and hydralazine therapy. *J.A.M.A.* 237:264–265, 1977.

Kelly, J. V.   Drugs used in the management of toxemia of pregnancy. *Clin. Obstet. Gynecol.* 20:395–410, 1977.

Koch-Weser, J.   Diazoxide. *N. Engl. J. Med.* 294:1271–1274, 1976.

Michael, C. A.   Intravenous diazoxide in the treatment of severe pre-eclamptic toxaemia and eclampsia. *Aust. N.Z. J. Obstet. Gynaecol.* 13:143–146, 1973.

Morris, J. A., Arce, J. J., Hamilton, C. J., Davidson, E. C., Maidman, J. E.,

Clark, J. H., Bloom, R. S. The management of severe pre-eclampsia and eclampsia with intravenous diazoxide. *Obstet. Gynecol.* 49:675–680, 1977.

Neurman, J., Weiss, B., Rabello, Y., Cabal, L., and Freeman, R. K. Diazoxide for the acute control of severe hypertension complicating pregnancy: A pilot study. *Obstet. Gynecol.* 53(Suppl.):50S–55S, 1979.

(RLB)

Digoxin (Lanoxin®)

INDICATIONS AND RECOMMENDATIONS

Digoxin is safe to use during pregnancy if the mother's blood levels are monitored frequently to avoid toxicity and to assure adequate digitalization. Digoxin is the most frequently prescribed of the digitalis glycosides, a group of drugs used in the treatment of congestive heart failure and atrial fibrillation, and in the prevention of paroxysmal atrial tachycardia.

SPECIAL CONSIDERATIONS IN PREGNANCY

Serum levels should be monitored in pregnant women near term to assure maintenance of therapeutic levels. Digoxin levels in the mother at term are usually significantly lower than levels taken several weeks postpartum on the same maintenance dose.

The digitalis glycosides readily cross the placenta. They seem to be preferentially concentrated in the fetal heart during the second half of pregnancy. Amniotic fluid levels of digoxin have been used to monitor fetal levels. Levels of the drug in the amniotic fluid slightly exceed those in fetal serum. Neonates and presumably the fetus seem to tolerate high serum levels of digoxin (2–4 μg/ml) much better than adults.

Digoxin is excreted in maternal milk. The total daily amount excreted, however, is far below the usual therapeutic dose for a newborn.

DOSAGE

The usual initial digitalizing dose is approximately 1.0 mg. This may be given orally or parenterally in several divided doses. The usual maintenance dose is approximately 0.25 mg per day. Serum levels must be monitored carefully to avoid toxicity. The therapeutic plasma levels are 0.5–2 ng/ml in adults. In some patients with atrial fibrillation, levels of 2.5–4 ng/ml may be required to slow the ventricular rate.

ADVERSE EFFECTS

Side effects of digoxin, which are rare when the drug is given in therapeutic doses include skin rashes, eosinophilia, and gynecomastia. Toxic effects of the digitalis derivatives include gastrointestinal symptoms of anorexia, nausea, and vomiting; visual changes; and alterations of cardiac rate and rhythm, especially extrasystoles and heart block. These toxic effects may be seen in patients with digoxin levels greater than 3 ng/ml. Digitalis toxicity can be potentiated by hypokalemia.

MECHANISM OF ACTION

The exact mechanism of action of digoxin is not known. The main pharmacological action of all digitalis glycosides is to increase the force and velocity of the myocardial contraction. They have a direct action on both the failing and nonfailing heart. When given to patients in congestive heart failure, cardiac output is increased, systolic emptying is more complete and end diastolic volumes and pressures are reduced. Sympathetic tone is reduced and in edematous patients diuresis results. Digitalis glycosides also decrease conduction velocity through the atrioventricular node. This effect is most apparent in patients with supraventricular tachyarrhythmias.

ABSORPTION AND BIOTRANSFORMATION

Approximately 65%–80% of an oral digoxin dose is absorbed. Only about 25% is bound to plasma proteins, and it is primarily excreted unchanged in the urine. The half-life of digoxin is approximately 36 hours and increases as renal function diminishes.

RECOMMENDED READING

Allonen, H., Kanto, J., and Iisalo, E.   The foeto-maternal distribution of digoxin in early human pregnancy. *Acta Pharmacol. Toxicol.* 39:477–480, 1976.

Rasmussen, R., Nawaz, M., and Steiness, E.   Mammary excretion of digoxin in goats. *Acta Pharmacol. Toxicol.* 36:377, 1975.

Rogers, M. C., Willerson, J. T., Goldblatt, A., and Smith, T. W.   Serum digoxin concentrations in the human fetus, neonate and infant. *N. Engl. J. Med.* 287:1010–1013, 1972.

Saarikoski, S.   Placental transfer and fetal uptake of ^{3}H digoxin in humans. *Br. J. Obstet. Gynaecol.* 83:879,884, 1976.

Seyka, L. F.   Digoxin: Placental transfer, effects on the fetus, and therapeutic use in the newborn. *Clin. Perinatol.* 2:23–35, 1975.

(TKM)

Dimenhydrinate (Dramamine®)

INDICATIONS AND RECOMMENDATIONS

Dimenhydrinate is contraindicated during pregnancy. It is an antihistamine used in the prevention and treatment of nausea and vomiting associated with motion sickness. The use of dimenhydrinate has been anecdotally associated with an increased incidence of premature labor. Meclizine is therefore preferable to this drug for the treatment of motion sickness during pregnancy.

RECOMMENDED READING

American Hospital Formulary Service. *Monograph for Dimenhydrinate.* Washington, D.C.: American Society of Hospital Pharmacists, May, 1977.

Goodman, L. S., and Gilman, A. *The Pharmacological Basis of Therapeutics* (5th ed.) New York: Macmillan, 1975. Pp. 608–611.

Long, J. W. *The Essential Guide to Prescription Drugs.* New York: Harper & Row, 1977. Pp. 250–251.

(DJK)

Diphenhydramine (Benadryl®)

INDICATIONS AND RECOMMENDATIONS

Diphenhydramine may be administered during pregnancy for the treatment of allergic disorders characterized by urticaria, pruritus, and rhinitis. It is the drug of choice for treatment of the oculogyric crisis resulting from phenothiazine administration and is useful in controlling other drug and blood transfusion reactions. Because of its possible association with an increased incidence of oral clefts, diphenhydramine should not be used in the first trimester for reducing self-limited symptoms and the discomfort of allergies. This drug is not recommended for use by nursing mothers since it may inhibit lactation; small amounts may be excreted in breast milk.

SPECIAL CONSIDERATIONS IN PREGNANCY

No prospective studies have been conducted that evaluate the safety of diphenhydramine's use during pregnancy. One large retrospective study, however, found no evidence incriminating this drug as a teratogen. In contrast with these findings, another, smaller, case-controlled study comparing groups of children with and without oral clefts found that the intake of diphenhydramine was significantly more frequent among the mothers of children with clefts. This was not true for mothers who had taken cyclizine.

DOSAGE

The usual oral dose is 50 mg taken three or four times a day. If parenteral administration is required, 10–50 mg may be given intravenously or by deep intramuscular injection. The maximum daily dosage is 400 mg.

ADVERSE EFFECTS

Anticholinergic side effects are most common; these include drowsiness, dry mouth and eyes, and, rarely, blurred vision. Anorexia, nausea, epigastric distress, and dizziness can also occur.

MECHANISM OF ACTION

Diphenhydramine is a competitive antagonist of histamine that decreases edema formation by diminishing capillary dilatation and permeability. It has anticholinergic activity and therefore reduces the tremor and rigidity of parkinsonism. It produces drowsiness and possesses local anesthetic ability when used topically.

ABSORPTION AND BIOTRANSFORMATION

Diphenhydramine is rapidly absorbed when taken orally or from sites of parenteral administration. When taken orally, the maximum effects are noted within 1 hour, and the duration of action is 4–6 hours, i.e., it reaches peak tissue concentrations in about 1 hour, and the tissues are almost depleted of the drug in about 6 hours. The main site of metabolic transformation is the liver, and excretion occurs via the kidney.

RECOMMENDED READING

Goodman, L. S., and Gilman, A. *The Pharmacological Basis of Therapeutics* (5th ed.). New York: Macmillan, 1975. Pp. 607–609.

Greenberger, P., and Patterson, R. Safety of therapy for allergic symptoms during pregnancy. *Ann. Intern. Med* 89:234–237, 1978.

Heinonen, O. P., Slone, D., and Shapiro, S. *Birth Defects and Drugs in Pregnancy*. Littleton, Mass.: Publishing Sciences Group, 1977. Pp. 323–334.

Nashimura, H., and Tanimura, T. *Aspects of the Teratogenicity of Drugs*. Amsterdam: Excerpta Medica, 1976.

Saxén, I. Cleft palate and maternal diphenhydramine intake. *Lancet* 1:407–408, 1974

(JRC)

Disopyramide (Norpace®)

INDICATIONS AND RECOMMENDATIONS

Disopyramide is relatively contraindicated during pregnancy because other therapeutic agents are preferable. This drug is an oral antiarrhythmic agent with electrophysiological actions similar to quinidine and procainamide. It is used in the treatment of premature ventricular contractions and episodes of ventricular tachycardia. Its use during pregnancy has been associated with the initiation of uterine contractions that subsided when the drug was discontinued. Therefore, if a class one antiarrhythmic is required during pregnancy, quinidine should be given.

RECOMMENDED READING

Befeler, B., Castellanos, A., Well, D. E., Vagueiro, M. C., and Yeh, B. K. Electrophysiologic effects of the antiarrhythmic agent disopyramide phosphate. *Am. J. Cardiol.* 35:282–287, 1975.

Leonard, R. F., Braun, T. E., and Levy, A. M. Initiation of uterine contractions by disopyramide during pregnancy. *N. Engl. J. Med.* 299:84–85, 1978.

(TKM)

Diuretics, Mercurial (Mercuhydrin®, Thiomerin®)

INDICATIONS AND RECOMMENDATIONS

Mercurial diuretics should not be used during pregnancy. In the rare instances when diuretics are needed to treat the pregnant woman (chronic hypertension, cardiogenic edema, chronic renal disease), other agents are preferable (the thiazide diuretics or furosemide). The diuretic effect of mercurial diuretics is caused by the intrarenal release of free mercury cations. These act on the tubular cell membranes to inhibit the reabsorption of sodium and chloride and the excretion of potassium. Classic symptoms of systemic mercury poisoning may follow the injudicious use of these agents, especially in patients with poor renal function.

Poisoning of the fetus by organic mercury has been well documented in the tragic "natural experiment" that took place in Japan in the early 1960s. Local fishermen who consumed methylmercury in shellfish caught in Minamata Bay developed a bizarre neurological syndrome. The methylmercury was traced to contamination of the bay by factory effluents. Affected individuals gave birth to congenitally anomalous babies with high perinatal mortality rates. Infants born to apparently asymptomatic mothers also developed cerebral palsy-like symptoms that varied in severity from mild spasticity to severe mental retardation and death. The type of compound used as a mercurial diuretic, however, was not implicated in this mercury poisoning syndrome.

RECOMMENDED READING

Goodman, L. S., and Gilman, A. *The Pharmacological Basis of Therapeutics* (5th ed.). New York: Macmillan, 1975. Pp. 823–825.

Joselow, M. M., Louria, D. B., and Browder, A. A. Mercurialism: Environmental and occupational aspects. *Ann. Intern. Med.* 76:119–130, 1972.

(RLB)

Diuretics, Thiazide: Chlorothiazide (Diuril®) and Hydrochlorothiazide (Hydrodiuril®)

INDICATIONS AND RECOMMENDATIONS

The use of the thiazides during pregnancy is controversial and if used at all, should be restricted to very specific situations. These drugs are diuretics and have antihypertensive activity in some patients with essential hypertension. The administration of thiazides does not prevent the development of preeclampsia-toxemia (PET), and these drugs have no role in the therapy of that condition. They also should not be used for the treatment of peripheral edema in the pregnant woman.

Since thiazides may decrease placental perfusion, controversy exists over the use of these drugs during pregnancy in patients with chronic hypertension. If started prior to conception, there is no strong evidence to suggest that continued therapy will compromise fetal growth. Some authors therefore recommend leaving a patient on this medication if it has been successfully used to control documented hypertension prior to the pregnancy. If, on the other hand, it becomes necessary to initiate treatment after the patient has become pregnant, the combination of a thiazide and methyldopa may reduce the potential for decreased placental perfusion. Some authors have recommended that the initiation of therapy with the thiazides be limited to the first half of pregnancy.

Frequent determinations of serum electrolytes should be made in pregnant women taking thiazide diuretics. Such women will frequently need oral potassium supplementation. Fetal growth should also be monitored closely throughout the period of therapy.

Thiazide diuretics may be given to breastfeeding mothers.

SPECIAL CONSIDERATIONS IN PREGNANCY

It is known that in PET many patients have a decreased intravascular volume. The administration of thiazides will reduce this further. Gant and colleagues have demonstrated a reduced metabolic clearance rate of dehydroepiandrosterone sulfate (MCR_{DS}) in 9 out of 10 pregnant women studied on the seventh day of thiazide therapy, which may represent decreased placental perfusion. These facts suggest that the administration of thiazides may compromise optimal fetal oxygenation and nutrition, especially in fetuses of patients with PET.

Additional problems that may occur when thiazides are given to pregnant women include maternal hyperuricemia. This rarely requires therapy but may mask the increase in serum uric acid that is often seen in association with developing PET. The thiazides cross the placenta and may cause symptomatic neonatal hyponatremia, hypokalemia, and thrombocytopenia.

The drugs are excreted in breast milk, but the amount of chlorothiazide that appears in the milk is probably too small to cause an adverse effect in the nursing infant.

DOSAGE

These drugs are usually given orally, with the diuretic effect occurring within 1 to 2 hours after absorption. The peak effect occurs in 4 hours and lasts about 6–12 hours. The two most commonly used thiazide diuretics are administered as follows:

	Minimal	*Usual*	*Maximal*
Chlorothiazide	500 mg qd	500 mg bid	750 mg bid
Hydrochlorothiazide	50 mg qd	50 mg bid	75 mg bid

ADVERSE EFFECTS

Side effects include hyponatremia, hypokalemia, and metabolic alkalosis. Hyperglycemia and allergic dermatitis with photosensitivity may occur. Occasionally pancreatitis, leukopenia, thrombocytopenia, and vasculitis may occur.

MECHANISM OF ACTION

The primary mode of action of thiazide diuretics is inhibition of electrolyte reabsorption in the distal tubules of the nephron. This results in an increase in sodium, chloride, and potassium excretion along with accompanying water. Uric acid excretion is also inhibited.

The thiazides cause an initial reduction in extracellular and plasma volume and a concurrent decrease in cardiac output. The effect is transient, and in 1 to 2 weeks the plasma volume and cardiac output return to normal levels, although a reduction in peripheral resistance is maintained. The persistent hypotensive effect may be secondary to either a direct action on the arteriolar smooth muscle or to changes of electrolyte concentration in the vessel wall. The latter could influence tone or pressor responsiveness. The autonomic reflexes essential for cardiovascular homeostasis are unimpaired. Plasma renin increases in response to sodium depletion and may remain increased throughout the time the drug is administered.

ABSORPTION AND BIOTRANSFORMATION

The thiazides are not metabolized in the body. They are rapidly absorbed from the gastrointestinal tract and distributed throughout the extracellular space and then are excreted unchanged in the urine.

RECOMMENDED READING

Gant, N. F., Madden, J. D., Siteri, P. K., MacDonald, P. C. The metabolic clearance rate of dehydroisoandrosterone sulfate: III. The effect of thiazide diuretics in normal and future pre-eclamptic pregnancy. *Am. J. Obstet. Gynecol.* 123:159–163, 1975.

Gifford, R. W., Jr. A guide to the practical use of diuretics. *J.A.M.A.* 235:1890–1893, 1976.

Goodman, L. S., and Gilman, A. *The Pharmacological Basis of Therapeutics* (5th ed.). New York: Macmillan, 1975. Pp. 828–833.

Krumlovsky, F. A., and delGreco, F. Diuretic agents: Mechanisms of action and clinical uses. *Postgrad. Med.* 59:105–110, 1976.

Pritchard, J. A. Standardized treatment of 154 consecutive cases of eclampsia. *Am. J. Obstet. Gynecol.* 123:543–552, 1975.

Pritchard, J. A., and MacDonald, P. *Williams Obstetrics* (15th ed.). New York: Appleton-Century-Crofts, 1976.

Werthmann, M. W., Jr., and Krees, S. V. Excretion of chlorothiazide in human breast milk. *J. Pediatr.* 81:781–783, 1972.

(RLB)

Docusates (over-the-counter):
(Colace®, Doxinate®, Surfak®)

INDICATIONS AND RECOMMENDATIONS

Dioctyl sulfosuccinates are safe to use during pregnancy. These drugs are used as stool softeners in people with hemorrhoids, anorectal disorders, hernias, and cardiovascular disease. They are widely used for women recovering from third and fourth degree perineal lacerations after delivery of their infants.

SPECIAL CONSIDERATIONS IN PREGNANCY

There are no special considerations to be kept in mind during pregnancy.

DOSAGE

Dioctyl sulfosuccinates vary in dosage from 50–480 mg/day taken by mouth. An effect is seen within 24–48 hours. Rectal preparations of 50–100 mg are also available.

ADVERSE EFFECTS

An overdose may cause anorexia, diarrhea, and vomiting.

MECHANISM OF ACTION

Dioctyl sulfosuccinates soften the fecal mass by lowering surface tension, thus facilitating penetration of water and fats.

ABSORPTION AND BIOTRANSFORMATION

They manifest no systemic effects because of their limited absorption, although a small portion is absorbed from the gastrointestinal tract and excreted in the bile.

RECOMMENDED READING

Goodman, L. S., and Gilman, A. *The Pharmacological Basis of Therapeutics* (5th ed.). New York: Macmillan, 1975. P. 977.

Nelson, M. M., and Forfar, J. O. Associations between drugs administered during pregnancy and congenital abnormalities of the fetus. *Br. Med. J.* 1:523–527, 1971.

Schenkel, B., and Vorherr, H. Non-prescription drugs during pregnancy: Potential teratogenic and toxic effects upon embryo and fetus. *J. Reprod. Med.* 12:27–45, 1974.

(RAC)

Doxylamine (Bendectin®, when combined with pyridoxine)

INDICATIONS AND RECOMMENDATIONS

Doxylamine is safe to use during pregnancy. Because of the extensive experience amassed, doxylamine in combination with pyridoxine (Bendectin®) is the drug of choice for relieving the nausea and vomiting associated with pregnancy.

SPECIAL CONSIDERATIONS IN PREGNANCY

Bendectin® is effective in relieving the nausea and vomiting associated with pregnancy. Large-scale studies of the use of doxylamine during pregnancy have failed to reveal teratogenic effects in humans.

A report in the *British Medical Journal* described 3 patients who took Debendox® (dicyclomine hydrochloride, 10 mg; doxylamine succinate, 10 mg; and pyridoxine hydrochloride, 10 mg) between 5½ and 6 weeks after their last menstrual periods and who gave birth to babies with a rare combination of anomalies. These deformities included extrusion of the abdominal contents and reduction deformity or total absence of a leg. This raised concern about the possible teratogenic effects on the fetus when the mother was exposed to this combination of drugs very early in gestation. In subsequent letters to the editor of the *British Medical Journal*, however, it was pointed out that identical cases of this uncommon, but not exceptionally rare, set of defects have occurred in women who had taken no drugs at all during the first trimester. Smithells and Sheppard have prospectively studied 372 mothers who had started taking Debendox® at 6 weeks of gestation or earlier. Of the offspring in this group, 1.9% had significant malformations, but none had gastroschisis or exomphalos. Of 1,620 mothers in the same study who started taking Debendox® at or before 12 weeks, 1.7% had malformed neonates. One infant whose mother had started taking Debendox at 12 weeks had exomphalos. There were no cases of gastroschisis. Therefore, there is currently no convincing evidence to incriminate this combination of drugs as a teratogen, even when taken early in pregnancy.

DOSAGE

Doxylamine is available in 10 mg tablets in combination with 10 mg of pyridoxine (Bendectin®). The usual dose of Bendectin® is 2 tablets hs. In severe cases, 1 additional tablet can be given in the morning and another in the afternoon.

ADVERSE EFFECTS

Side effects can include drowsiness, vertigo, nervousness, epigastric pain, headache, palpitation, diarrhea, and disorientation.

MECHANISM OF ACTION

Doxylamine's antinauseant effect appears to be due to an inhibition of vestibular stimulation and conduction. It is also an antihistamine that acts by competitive inhibition at the H_1 receptor.

ABSORPTION AND BIOTRANSFORMATION

Doxylamine is readily absorbed from the gastrointestinal tract and is widely distributed throughout the body. It appears to be metabolized in the liver.

RECOMMENDED READING

Biggs, J. S. G.   Vomiting in pregnancy: Causes and management. *Drugs* 9:299–306, 1975.

Check, W. A.   CDC study: No evidence for teratogenicity of Bendectin. *J.A.M.A.* 242:2518, 1979.

Donnai, D., and Harris, R.   Unusual fetal malformations after antiemetics in early pregnancy. *Br. Med. J.* 691–692, April 22, 1978.

Heinonen, O. P., Slone, D., and Shapiro, S.   *Birth Defects and Drugs in Pregnancy*. Littleton, Mass.: Publishing Sciences Group, 1977. Pp. 323–334.

Henderson, I.   Congenital deformities associated with Bendectin. *CMA Journal* 117:721–722, 1977.

Kohn, A., and Parsons, A.   Fetal malformation not associated with Debendox. (Letter to editor). *Br. Med. J.* 1216, May 6, 1978.

Long, J. W.   *The Essential Guide to Prescription Drugs* (1st ed.). New York: Harper & Row, 1977. Pp. 265–267.

Mellor, S.   Fetal malformation after Debendox treatment in early pregnancy (Letter to editor). *Br. Med. J.* 1055, April 22, 1978.

Milkovich, L., VandenBerg, B. J.   An evaluation of the teratogenicity of certain antinauseant drugs. *Am. J. Obstet. Gynecol.* 125:244–248, 1976.

Smithells, R. W., and Sheppard, S.   Letter to editor. *Br. Med. J.* 1055, April 22, 1978.

(DJK)

Ephedrine

INDICATIONS AND RECOMMENDATIONS

The use of ephedrine during pregnancy should be limited to the correction of maternal hypotension unresponsive to rapid fluid infusion and left lateral uterine displacement following the administration of a spinal or epidural anesthetic. This drug should not be used to treat asthma in the pregnant woman as other agents for that purpose are preferable.

SPECIAL CONSIDERATIONS IN PREGNANCY

There is no information available as to whether the drug crosses the placenta, is secreted in breast milk, or whether it has teratogenic effects. Administration to normal pregnant ewes does not decrease uterine blood flow, alter fetal acid-base status, or produce changes in fetal heart rate. When ephedrine is used in combination with oxytocics, severe hypertension may develop. It must be used with extreme caution in patients with chronic hypertension or toxemia.

DOSAGE

For the treatment of hypotension, ephedrine is administered intravenously in 10–20 mg doses every 60 seconds as needed to keep the systolic blood pressure above 100 mm Hg. It is rarely necessary to use more than 60 mg for this purpose. Its duration of action is several hours.

ADVERSE EFFECTS

Side effects associated with the use of ephedrine include hypertension, cardiac arrhythmias, palpitations, insomnia, tremor, and anxiety.

MECHANISM OF ACTION

Ephedrine has both alpha and beta adrenergic actions. It acts by stimulating the release of stored norepinephrine and by direct stimulation of adrenergic receptors.

The effects of ephedrine in the body are widespread. Because it produces mild bronchodilatation, it has therefore been used as an adjunct to theophylline therapy in asthma. It increases both systolic and diastolic blood pressures and decreases pulse pressure; heart rate is generally unchanged; cardiac output is increased; renal and splanchnic blood flow are decreased; and coronary, cerebral, and muscle blood flow are increased. Ephedrine decreases uterine activity (β_2 effect). It also produces mydriasis when applied topically.

ABSORPTION AND BIOTRANSFORMATION

Ephedrine is well absorbed when given orally. Most of the drug is metabolized by deamination and conjugation. Both metabolites and unchanged drug are excreted in the urine.

RECOMMENDED READING

Chen, K. K., and Schmidt, C. F.   Ephedrine and related substances. *Medicine* 9:1–117, 1930.

Eng, M., Berges, P. V., and Ueland, K.   The effects of methoxamine and ephedrine in normotensive pregnant primates. *Anesthesia* 35:354–360, 1970.

Ralstow, D. H., Schnider, S. M., and deLorimier, A. A.   Effect of equipotent doses of ephedrine, metaraminol, mephentermine, and methoxamine on uterine blood flow in the pregnant ewe. *Anesthesia* 40:354–370, 1974.

Schnider, S. M., DeLorimier, A. A., and Holl, J. W.   Vasopressor in obstetrics: I. Correction of fetal acidosis with ephedrine during spinal hypotension. *Am. J. Obstet. Gynecol.* 102:911–919, 1968.

Weinberger, M.   Use of ephedrine in bronchodilator therapy. *Pediatr. Clin. North Am.* 22:121–127, 1975.

(RJR)

Ergonovine Maleate (Ergotrate®)

INDICATIONS AND RECOMMENDATIONS

Ergonovine maleate is contraindicated during pregnancy prior to delivery of the infant. Its use is indicated for the prevention and treatment of postpartum and postabortal hemorrhage due to uterine atony. It may also be used during the puerperium to promote involution of the uterus. It is a direct stimulant of gravid and nongravid uterine muscle, although the gravid uterus is much more sensitive to its effects. Due to the high degree of uterine stimulation produced, ergonovine is not recommended for antepartum use, nor should it be administered prior to delivery of the placenta. It should not be used for the induction or augmentation of labor because of its tendency to produce tetanic contractions.

Several studies have shown ergonovine to interfere with normal secretion of prolactin in the immediate puerperium. Lactation thus may be delayed or inhibited in nursing mothers when it has been administered.

RECOMMENDED READING

Canales, R., Garrudo, F., Zarate, A., Mason, M., and Soria, J.   Effect of ergonovine on prolactin secretion and milk letdown. *Obstet. Gynecol.* 48:228–229, 1976.

Chase, G., Deno, R., Gennaro, A., et al., (Eds.).   *Remington's Pharmaceutical Sciences* (14th ed.). Easton, Pa.: Mack Publishing, 1970. Pp. 951–952.

Floss, H., Cassidy, J., and Robbers, J.   Influence of ergot alkaloids on pituitary prolactin and prolactin-dependent processes. *J. Pharm. Sci.* 62:699–715, 1973.

Goodman, L. S., and Gilman, A.   *The Pharmacological Basis of Therapeutics* (5th ed.). New York: Macmillan, 1975. Pp. 540–541, 872–879.

Reis, R. A., Gerbie, A. B., and Gerbie, M. V.   Reducing hazards of the newborn during cesarean section. *Obstet. Gynecol.* 46:676–678, 1975.

(PLR)

Ergotamine Tartrate (Gynergen®; Ergomar®; Ergostat®; Cafergot®, with caffeine)

INDICATIONS AND RECOMMENDATIONS

Ergotamine tartrate is contraindicated during pregnancy. This drug, which is used to abort migraine and cluster headaches, produces alpha-adrenergic blockade and more importantly acts on the central nervous system and directly stimulates smooth muscle.

It should not be used during pregnancy because it can create tetanic uterine contractions. It may also cause a significant increase in blood pressure at therapeutic doses. Administration of this drug during organogenesis has produced an increased incidence of fetal wastage in rats and fetal growth retardation in rats, mice, and rabbits. No human studies are available.

RECOMMENDED READING

AMA Drug Evaluations (3rd ed.). Littleton, Mass.: Publishing Sciences Group, 1977. Pp. 358–359.

American Hospital Formulary Service. *Monograph for Ergotamine Tartrate.* Section 12:16. Washington, D.C.: American Society of Hospital Pharmacists, 1959.

Floss, H., Cassidy, J., and Robbers, J.   Influence of ergot alkaloids on pituitary prolactin and prolactin-dependent processes. *J. Pharm. Sci.* 62:699–715, 1973.

Goodman, L. S., and Gilman, A.   *The Pharmacological Basis of Therapeutics* (5th ed.). New York: Macmillan, 1975. Pp. 540–541, 872–878.

Grauwiler, J., and Schön, H.   Teratological experiments with ergotamine in mice, rats and rabbits. *Teratology* 7:227–236, 1973.

Parkes, J. Relief of pain—headache, facial neuralgia, migraine and phantom limbs. *Br. Med. J.* 4:282–289, 1975.

(PLR)

Erythromycin (E-mycin®, Erythrocin®)

INDICATIONS AND RECOMMENDATIONS

Erythromycin is safe to use during pregnancy. It is an antibiotic used to treat gram-positive infections and syphilis in penicillin-allergic patients. It is also effective against gonococci, *Hemophilus* species, the organism of Legionnaires' disease, and large viruses of the lymphogranuloma venereum group.

SPECIAL CONSIDERATIONS IN PREGNANCY

Fetal plasma concentrations are 5–20% of those found in maternal plasma. This drug is safe for the fetus and is often recommended to treat syphilis in penicillin-allergic pregnant women. Its efficacy in fetal syphilis is questionable.

DOSAGE

The usual oral dose is 250–500 mg every 6 hours. Parenteral administration is rarely indicated. When given intravenously, it is preferable that erythromycin be administered in a continuous drip rather than being pulsed. The usual intravenous or intramuscular dose is 1–4 gm/day.

ADVERSE EFFECTS

Occasional side effects include stomatitis and gastrointestinal disturbance. Cholestatic hepatitis has been reported when erythromycin estolate is given to adults. Allergic reactions and transient deafness are rare side effects. Because of the potentially serious hepatic effects, erythromycin estolate should not be used.

MECHANISM OF ACTION

Erythromycin is an orally effective macrolide antibiotic that inhibits protein synthesis by binding to 50S ribosomal subunits of sensitive microorganisms.

ABSORPTION AND BIOTRANSFORMATION

Erythromycin is well absorbed orally. The stearate is broken down in acid and is administered in acid-resistant capsules. The estolate is less susceptible to acid degradation. Erythromycin is concentrated in the liver and excreted in bile. Only 2%–5% of the oral dose is excreted by the kidneys, while 12%–15% appears in the urine following intravenous infusion.

RECOMMENDED READING

Handbook of Antimicrobial Therapy. The Medical Letter on Drugs and Therapeutics (Rev. ed.), 1978.

Philipson, A., Sabath, L. D., and Charles, D. Transplacental passage of erythromycin and clindamycin. *N. Engl. J. Med.* 288:1219–1221, 1973.

(GRD)

Estrogens (Synthetic and natural)

INDICATIONS AND RECOMMENDATIONS

Both steroidal and nonsteroidal estrogens are contraindicated during pregnancy. In the past the nonsteroidal estrogens have been prescribed for maintenance of diabetic pregnancies and the prevention of spontaneous abortions.

Maternal side effects may include nausea, vomiting, skin changes, thrombophlebitis, pulmonary embolization, and cholestatic jaundice. Important fetal effects have been noted when nonsteroidal estrogen (specifically diethylstilbestrol [DES]) was administered during the first trimester. These include an increased incidence of adenocarcinoma and adenosis of the vagina, uterine deformity, and perhaps squamous cell cancers in females. Testicular cysts and oligospermia have been noted when developing male gonadal tissue has been exposed to these compounds in utero. The estrogens are secreted in breast milk.

It is recommended that estrogens, both steroidal and nonsteroidal, natural and synthetic, not be utilized in pregnancy. There is no proof that they are beneficial, and there is good evidence that the nonsteroidal estrogens may produce fetal genital tract anomalies and disease.

RECOMMENDED READING

Bibbo, N., Gill, W. B., Azizi, F., Blough, R., Fang, V. S., Rosenfield, R. L., Schumacher, G. F. B., Sleeper, K., Sonek, M. G., and Wied, G. L. Follow up study of male and female offspring of DES exposed mothers. *Obstet. Gynecol.* 49:1–8, 1977.

Herbst, A. L., Kurman, R. J., and Scully, R. E. Vaginal and cervical abnormalities after exposure to stilbestrol in utero. *Obstet. Gynecol.* 30:287–298, 1972.

Kaufman, R. H., Binder, G. L., Gray, P. M., and Adam, E. Upper genital tract changes associated with exposure in utero to diethylstilbestrol. *Am. J. Obstet. Gynecol.* 128:51–59, 1977.

(AHD)

Ethacrynic Acid (Edecrin®)

INDICATIONS AND RECOMMENDATIONS

The use of ethacrynic acid is relatively contraindicated during pregnancy because other therapeutic agents are preferable. It is a loop diuretic with activity similar to that of furosemide. The major complications associated with the use of ethacrynic acid in pregnancy are ototoxicity and hypokalemic alkalosis. These sequelae have been observed both in pregnant women and their offspring. It should be noted, however, that reports describing the uneventful use of this drug during pregnancy have been published. If a loop diuretic is indicated for an obstetrical patient, furosemide is the drug of choice.

RECOMMENDED READING

Finnerty, F. A. Hypertension in pregnancy. *Clin. Obstet. Gynecol.* 18:145–154, 1975.

Fort, A. T., Morrison, J. C., and Fish, S. A. Iatrogenic hypokalemia of pregnancy by furosemide and ethacrynic acid. *J. Reprod. Med.* 6:207–208, 1971.

Harrison, K. A. Ethacrynic acid in blood transfusion—its effects on plasma volume and urine flow in severe anaemia in pregnancy. *Br. Med. J.* 4:84–86, 1968.

Jones, H. C. Intrauterine ototoxicity—a case report and review of the literature. *J. Natl. Med. Assoc.* 65:201–203, 1973.

Schneider, W. J., and Becker, E. L. Acute transient hearing loss after ethacrynic acid. *Arch. Intern. Med.* 117:715–717, 1966.

Young, B. K., and Haft, J. I. Treatment of pulmonary edema with ethacrynic acid during labor. *Am. J. Obstet. Gynecol.* 107:330–331, 1970.

(JAG)

Ethchlorvynol (Placidyl®)

INDICATIONS AND RECOMMENDATIONS

The use of ethchlorvynol is relatively contraindicated during pregnancy because other therapeutic agents are preferable. It is used primarily as a hypnotic agent in the treatment of insomnia. This drug offers no therapeutic advantage over barbiturate or nonbarbiturate sedatives. Little is known about its effects on the pregnant woman or fetus. In dogs, it has been shown to achieve significant fetal blood levels within 90 minutes after maternal ingestion. Symptoms resembling congenital narcotic withdrawal have been described in the human newborn after the mother has ingested ethchlorvynol.

No sedative has been found to be absolutely safe during pregnancy as most cross the placenta and produce sedation and withdrawal symptoms in the newborn. Should such therapy be required during pregnancy, phenobarbital may be used (see *Phenobarbital*).

RECOMMENDED READING

Goodman, L. S., and Gilman, A.   *The Pharmacological Basis of Therapeutics* (5th ed.). New York: Macmillan, 1975. Pp. 129–130.

Hume, A. S., Williams, J. M., and Douglas, B. H.   Disposition of ethchlorvynol in maternal blood, fetal blood, amniotic fluid and chorionic fluid. *J. Reprod. Med.* 6:229–231, 1971.

Rumack, B. H., and Walravens, P. A.   Neonatal withdrawal following maternal ingestion of ethchlorvynol. *Pediatrics* 52:714–716, 1973.

(CET)

Ethosuximide (Zarontin®)

INDICATIONS AND RECOMMENDATIONS

Ethosuximide may be administered to pregnant women in the treatment of petit mal epilepsy. This condition is rare in women of child-bearing age and its effects upon the fetus have not been studied in depth. If a woman's petit mal epilepsy persists during her child-bearing years and requires treatment, therapy with ethosuximide may be continued through pregnancy.

SPECIAL CONSIDERATIONS IN PREGNANCY

The placental transfer of ethosuximide has been demonstrated in rats; fetal and maternal tissue levels appear to be similar. There is no information regarding adverse effects of this drug on human pregnancy.

Although ethosuximide is detectable in breast milk, the amount has never been quantified; pharmacological effects on infants being breast-fed have not been described.

DOSAGE

The starting dose should be 20 mg/kg/day, which produces a plasma level of approximately 60 μg/ml. The usual maintenance dose is 20–40 mg/kg/day. Since petit mal seizures usually occur in the early part of the day, it is preferable to divide the daily total dose into three to four portions and to give the last one not later than 6 P.M.

ADVERSE EFFECTS

Dose-related side effects include drowsiness, headache, hiccough, euphoria, and disequilibrium. Ethosuximide may cause local irritative effects on the stomach, with anorexia, gastric discomfort, nausea, and vomiting. Non-dose-related effects include rash, Stevens-Johnson syndrome, a lupus-like syndrome, and, rarely, leukopenia, pancytopenia, aplastic anemia, and changes in personality and intellect.

MECHANISM OF ACTION

The chemical mode of action of ethosuximide has not been extensively explored. It has been found to raise the brain-to-blood glucose ratio in mice. This finding suggests that the drug facilitates the transport of glucose from blood to brain. It also decreases the concentration of Krebs' cycle intermediates in the brain.

Ethosuximide has a direct depressant effect on the cortex of the brain and elevates the threshold for electroshock-induced seizures. It suppresses the paroxysmal three cycles per second spike-and-wave activity associated with absence seizures. It is not effective in the treatment of grand mal seizures.

ABSORPTION AND BIOTRANSFORMATION

Absorption is fairly rapid and complete from the alimentary tract, with peak plasma levels occurring 1 to 4 hours after a single oral dose. It has been demonstrated that ethosuximide is absorbed faster from a syrup preparation than from capsules. It is fairly uniformly distributed throughout the body, except for adipose tissue in which levels are lower than elsewhere. The drug is minimally bound to plasma and spinal fluid proteins. Plasma concentrations of 40–100 μg/ml appear to have the best correlation with control of petit mal epilepsy. Ten to twenty percent of ethosuximide is excreted unchanged in the urine. The remaining drug is metabolized in the liver.

RECOMMENDED READING

Eadie, M. J., and Tyrer, J. H. *Anticonvulsant Therapy*. Edinburgh: Churchill-Livingstone, 1974.
Goodman, L. S., Gilman, A. *The Pharmacological Basis of Therapeutics* (5th ed.). New York: Macmillan, 1975. Pp. 212–213, 220–221.
Woodbury, D. M., Penry, J. K., and Schmidt, R. P. *Antiepileptic* Drugs. New York: Raven Press, 1972.

(EMT)

Furosemide (Lasix®)

INDICATIONS AND RECOMMENDATIONS

Furosemide may be administered to pregnant women for the treatment of congestive heart failure and some cases of chronic renal disease. It is an extremely powerful saluretic that may rapidly decrease maternal intravascular volume and, consequently, diminish uteroplacental perfusion. For this reason, it must be used with extreme care in the obstetric patient. It is not indicated for the routine treatment of hypertension or peripheral edema during pregnancy.

SPECIAL CONSIDERATIONS IN PREGNANCY

Furosemide must be administered with great caution in the pregnant patient. As indicated above, hypovolemia may lead to decreased uterine blood flow, which can affect the fetus adversely. If the drug is used, the fetus should be carefully monitored for evidence of intrauterine compromise.

Animal studies have shown furosemide to cause unexplained maternal deaths and abortions in rabbits as well as an increased incidence of fetal hydronephrosis in rats. In humans, furosemide crosses the placenta and increases the ultrasonically measured hourly fetal urinary production rate. It can also increase fetal serum and amniotic fluid uric acid levels.

DOSAGE

Furosemide may be given intravenously or orally in the following range:

	Minimum	Usual	Maximum
Oral	20 mg qd	40 mg qd–qid	600 mg daily
Intravenous	10 mg/dose	20–40 mg/dose	600 mg daily

ADVERSE EFFECTS

The most serious side effect of furosemide is severe hypovolemia. Hyponatremia, hypokalemia, hypochloremia, hyperuricemia, and metabolic alkalosis may also occur. Glucose intolerance, hearing loss, and interstitial nephritis have been reported. Occasionally, skin rash, paresthesias, gastrointestinal disturbances, thrombocytopenia, and neutropenia are seen.

MECHANISM OF ACTION

Furosemide acts directly on the ascending limb of the loop of Henle. It works primarily by inhibiting sodium and chloride reabsorption in the loop. In the normally functioning kidney, furosemide causes excretion of 30–40% of the filtered sodium load and produces a prompt diuresis where maximal sodium and water reabsorption has not already taken place in the proximal tubule. The drug's effectiveness decreases as the glomerular filtration rate approaches 20 ml/min.

ABSORPTION AND BIOTRANSFORMATION

Furosemide is readily absorbed from the gastrointestinal tract and is strongly bound to plasma proteins. Two-thirds of an oral dose is excreted in the urine, the remainder being eliminated via the feces. Urinary excretion is accomplished by both glomerular filtration and proximal tubular secretion. Only a small fraction of the drug is metabolized.

RECOMMENDED READING

Gant, N. F. The metabolic clearance rate of dehydroisoandrosterone sulfate: III. The effect of thiazide diuretics in normal and future pre-eclamptic pregnancies. *Am. J. Obstet. Gynecol.* 123:159–163, 1975.

Gifford, R. W., Jr. A guide to the practical use of diuretics. *J.A.M.A.* 235:1890–1893, 1976.

Goodman, L. S., and Gilman, A. *The Pharmacological Basis of Therapeutics* (5th ed.). New York: Macmillan, 1975. Pp. 833–836.

Krunlovsky, F. A., and del Grew, C. Diuretic agents: Mechanism of action and clinical uses. *Postgrad. Med.* 59:105–110, 1976.

Pritchard, J. A. Standardized treatment of 154 consecutive cases of eclampsia. *Am. J. Obstet. Gynecol.* 123:543–552, 1975.

Pritchard, J. A., and MacDonald, P. *Williams Obstetrics* (15th ed.). New York: Appleton-Century-Crofts, 1976.

(PCL)

Gamma Benzene Hexachloride (Lindane) (Kwell®)

INDICATIONS AND RECOMMENDATIONS

Gamma benzene hexachloride may be administered to pregnant women for the treatment of scabies and lice. Head lice (*Pediculosis capitis*) and crab lice (*Phthirus pubis*) are treated with the cream, lotion, and shampoo forms of the drug. Scabies (*Sarcoptes scabiei*) are treated with the cream and lotion forms. Treatment should be such that only a minimal amount of drug is absorbed percutaneously.

SPECIAL CONSIDERATIONS IN PREGNANCY

There have thus far been no reports of fetal malformation associated with the use of gamma benzene hexachloride by the pregnant woman. In order to minimize the amount of drug absorbed, however, it is recommended that the lotion or cream be applied to dry, cool skin, that in the treatment of scabies the product be allowed to remain on the skin for only 8 hours, and that pediculosis be treated with the shampoo.

DOSAGE

In the treatment of scabies a thin layer of the cream or lotion should be applied to the entire skin surface. It should be allowed to remain on the skin for 8 hours and then the skin should be washed thoroughly. A second or third application may be made at weekly intervals if necessary.

In the treatment of pediculosis, the affected and surrounding hairy areas should be wet with 30 ml of shampoo. Water should then be added and the shampoo worked into a lather for at least 4 minutes. The area should then be rinsed thoroughly and dried with a towel. A fine-tooth comb should be used to remove any remaining nit shells. If necessary, the treatment may be repeated in 24 hours but not more than twice in 1 week.

ADVERSE EFFECTS

Side effects are rare but may be dangerous when they occur. Fatal cases of aplastic anemia have resulted from prolonged exposure to the vaporized drug. In addition, very high doses applied percutaneously or taken orally have produced convulsions in humans.

MECHANISM OF ACTION

The mechanism of action of gamma benzene hexachloride is similar to that of DDT. It is absorbed through the exoskeletons of many arthropods and acts directly on their nervous tissue to produce convulsions and death. It is an excellent miticide and pediculocide that produces relief of symptoms usually within 24 hours of application.

ABSORPTION AND BIOTRANSFORMATION

The exact pharmacokinetics of gamma benzene hexachloride are unknown. One study, however, reported recovery of 9.3% of the dose in the urine after a 24-hour application to unwashed skin. In animals it appears that absorption is greater through the skin of the young.

RECOMMENDED READING

Gamma benzene hexachloride (Kwell and other products) alert. *FDA Drug Bull.* 6:28, 1976.

Goodman, L. S., and Gilman, A. *The Pharmacological Basis of Therapeutics* (5th ed.). New York: Macmillan, 1975. Pp. 1014–1015.

Lee, B., and Groth, P. Scabies: Transcutaneous poisoning during treatment. *Pediatrics* 59:643, 1977.

(TKM)

Griseofulvin (Fulvicin-U/F®, Grifulvin V®, Grisactin®)

INDICATIONS AND RECOMMENDATIONS

Griseofulvin use is contraindicated during pregnancy. It is a systemic agent used to treat fungal infections of the skin, hair, and nails. Such infections are not life-threatening and since griseofulvin is a known teratogen in laboratory animals and has been demonstrated to cross the human placenta, its use is therefore contraindicated during pregnancy. Its use should be postponed until after delivery.

RECOMMENDED READING

Goodman, L. S., and Gilman, A. *The Pharmacological Basis of Therapeutics* (5th ed.). New York: Macmillan, 1975. Pp. 1239–1241.

Klein, M. F., and Beall, J. R. Griseofulvin: A teratogenic study. *Science* 175:1483–1484, 1972.

Kucers, A., and Bennet, N. *The Use of Antibiotics* (2nd ed.). London: William Heinemann Medical Books, 1975.

Rubin, A., and Dvornik, D. Placental transfer of griseofulvin. *Am. J. Obstet. Gynecol.* 92:882–883, 1965.

(TKM)

Guanethidine (Ismelin®)

INDICATIONS AND RECOMMENDATIONS

Guanethidine is contraindicated during pregnancy. This drug is a powerful postganglionic sympatholytic compound and may be used as an antihypertensive agent. It acts by blocking norepinephrine release from nerve endings, which exposes more of the neurotransmitter to metabolic inactivation within the neuron and results in a depletion of the storage pool.

Many of the observed side effects of guanethidine are due to the combination of adrenergic inhibition and unopposed parasympathetic function. Adverse effects include significant orthostatic and exercise hypotension, bradycardia, increased gastric secretion, and frequent bowel movements or diarrhea.

Experience with guanethidine in the pregnant woman is limited, and its effects on the fetus are unknown. Pronounced postural hypotension and other annoying sequelae of this drug make it a poor choice for the therapy of hypertension in pregnancy. Guanethidine appears in breast milk in very small quantities and can probably be given to nursing mothers.

RECOMMENDED READING

Goodman, L. S., and Gilman, A. *The Pharmacological Basis of Therapeutics* (5th ed.). New York: Macmillan, 1975. Pp. 553–556.

Kelly, J. V. Drugs used in the management of toxemia of pregnancy. *Clin. Obstet. Gynecol.* 20:395–410, 1977.

(PCL)

Haloperidol (Haldol®)

INDICATIONS AND RECOMMENDATIONS

Haloperidol may be administered to pregnant women for the chronic treatment of psychosis. This agent is similar to the phenothiazines and is used to treat delusions, hallucinations, disordered thought processes, paranoid symptoms, and withdrawal psychoses. It has also been reported to be effective in the treatment of Gilles de la Tourette's disease. Because of isolated case reports of teratogenicity, haloperidol use in pregnancy should be limited to those psychotic patients who require long-term medication.

Haloperidol will calm the excited patient and induce sleep. It will block apomorphine-induced emesis.

SPECIAL CONSIDERATIONS IN PREGNANCY

Congenital anomalies including phocomelia have been reported in infants whose mothers have taken haloperidol during pregnancy. The data, however, are insufficient to implicate haloperidol as the only contributor to the malformations.

Due to the pharmacological similarities of this drug to the phenothiazines, fetal and neonatal responses to maternal administration may be similar. Haloperidol is excreted in breast milk, but to date there are no reports of adverse effects in human infants nursed by mothers taking this drug.

DOSAGE

The usual dosage is between 0.5 and 2 mg two to three times a day. Some patients given long-term treatment are drug-resistant and may require 3–5 mg two to three times a day. In rare cases haloperidol has been used in doses in excess of 100 mg daily.

ADVERSE EFFECTS

Haloperidol can cause galactorrhea. Its autonomic effects are less prominent than other antipsychotic drugs. The most frequent side effects are extrapyramidal symptoms, akathisia dystonia, dry mouth, and constipation. Occasional side effects include blood dyscrasias, hypotension, drowsiness, and menstrual changes. Rare side effects are cholestatic jaundice, photosensitivity, and convulsions.

MECHANISM OF ACTION

The mechanism of action of haloperidol is only partly known and is thought to be similar to that of the phenothiazines. Its effects may be due to blockage of dopamine receptors in the caudate nucleus and inhibition of the activation of adenyl cyclase by dopamine.

ABSORPTION AND BIOTRANSFORMATION

Haloperidol is readily absorbed from the gastrointestinal tract. The drug is concentrated in the liver with about 15% of a dose excreted in the bile. About 40% is excreted in the urine during the first 5 days after a single dose.

RECOMMENDED READING

AMA Drug Evaluations (3rd ed.). Littleton, Mass.: Publishing Sciences Group, 1977. Pp. 420–451, 1090–1105.

American Hospital Formulary Service. *Monograph on Haloperidol. Section 28:16.08.* Washington, D.C.: American Society of Hospital Pharmacists, March, 1972.

Ayd, F. J., Jr. Excretion of psychotropic drugs in human breast milk. *Int. Drug Ther. Newslett.* 8:33–40, 1973.

Baldessarini, R. J. *Chemotherapy in Psychiatry.* Cambridge: Harvard University Press, 1977. Pp. 12–56.

Drugs for psychiatric disorders. *Med. Lett. Drugs Ther.* 18:89–96, 1976.

Goodman, L. S., and Gilman, A. *The Pharmacological Basis of Therapeutics* (5th ed.). New York: Macmillan, 1975. Pp. 152–174.

(CRS)

Heparin

INDICATIONS AND RECOMMENDATIONS

Heparin is safe to use during pregnancy. It is the anticoagulant of choice during the first and third trimesters. While some researchers have recommended use of oral anticoagulants during the second trimester in selected patients, intravenous or subcutaneous heparin is *probably* the drug of choice throughout pregnancy.

Anticoagulants are indicated in the treatment and prophylaxis of pulmonary embolism, venous thromboembolic disease, atrial fibrillation with embolization; prevention of clotting in arterial and cardiac surgery; and the prevention of clotting with implanted prosthetic devices such as heart valves. The use of heparin to treat disseminated intravascular coagulation (DIC) of obstetric origin remains controversial.

When initiated prior to elective surgery, a course of heparin given subcutaneously and in subtherapeutic doses has been reported to be effective in preventing postoperative deep vein phlebitis. "Minidose" therapy has also been given as prophylaxis against phlebitis in obese patients confined to bed for prolonged periods and in women with a history of deep vein problems in prior pregnancies.

Patients being fully anticoagulated with heparin may require continuous hospitalization throughout the course of the therapy, although selected individuals can be instructed to give their own intravenous or subcutaneous injections with outpatient monitoring. Minidose heparin prophylaxis can be given entirely on an outpatient basis with periodic monitoring. Heparin can be given to breastfeeding mothers.

SPECIAL CONSIDERATIONS IN PREGNANCY

No unusual maternal effects have been reported. Since the drug does not cross the placenta, it has no direct effect on the fetus. Heparin given to breastfeeding women does not have any demonstrable ill effect on the nursing infant.

Effective treatment of DIC rests with the recognition and adequate eradication of the underlying illness. To date, no controlled double-blind prospective study has demonstrated a beneficial effect of the use of heparin in treating DIC of obstetric origin. Moreover, its use has been reported to be deleterious rather than helpful in some cases.

DOSAGE

The anticoagulant potency of a given weight of heparin may vary from one preparation to another. It should always be ordered in USP units as opposed to cubic centimeters of solution. The effect is variable among patients, and the dose therefore must be monitored with either Lee-White whole blood clotting time or activated partial thromboplastin times (APTT). The Lee-White time should be two and one-half to three times control values, and the APTT time should be one and one-half to two and one-half times control values. Requirements for heparin may dramatically decrease as the thrombophlebitic process is brought under control.

Table 6 gives the frequency and dose of heparin used with each method of administration. Continuous infusion is the preferred method of administration. There are fewer bleeding complications and monitoring is simplified. With this type of infusion, too, blood may be drawn at any time, while blood for clotting studies must be drawn immediately prior to the next dose when intermittent schedules are used.

In the case of overdose, heparin is immediately discontinued. If it is felt necessary to reverse the anticoagulant effect, protamine sulfate is administered as a 1% solution in a dose of 1 mg for each 100 units of heparin thought to be present at the time of neutralization. (Consider 30 minutes to be the half-life of IV heparin, and 60 minutes the half-life of SC heparin.) If protamine is given in excess,

Table 6. Heparin Administration: Method, Frequency, Dose

Method of Administration	Frequency	Dose (units)
Full heparinization		
Subcutaneous	Initial dose	10,000
	q8h	8,000–10,000
	q12h	12,000–20,000
Intermittent IV	Initial dose	10,000
	q4h	5,000–10,000
Continuous IV	Continuous	5,000 (loading)
		20,000–40,000/day
Prophylactic preoperative miniheparinization		
Subcutaneous	q8–12h (begin the night before surgery)	5,000

Note: Some authorities suggest giving 5,000 units of heparin subcutaneously every 12–24 hours for outpatient prophylaxis in patients with a history of deep vein phlebitis in a prior pregnancy. These patients should be monitored with APTT's every 3–4 weeks.

it may itself act as an anticoagulant by interfering with the action of thrombin on fibrinogen. Some clinicians therefore will give half of the projected dose and observe the effect on the APTT.

ADVERSE EFFECTS

The most important side effect associated with heparin administration is hemorrhage in the mother. The anticoagulant action of this substance can be rapidly reversed with protamine sulfate. The following conditions have been considered by some authors to be contraindications to the use of heparin:

1. Any condition in which an increased bleeding tendency exists
2. Subacute bacterial endocarditis
3. Acute pericarditis
4. Threatened abortion
5. Suspected intracranial bleeding

Hypersensitivity reactions are usually manifested by chills, fever, and urticaria, but true anaphylactoid reactions have also occurred. Unusual side effects include transient alopecia, reversible thrombocytopenia, and rebound hyperlipemia when the drug is discontinued. Osteoporosis and suppression of renal function have been reported when the drug has been used for over 6 months.

When given simultaneously with heparin, the following drugs may cause excessive bleeding: aspirin and aspirin derivatives, phenylbutazone, indomethacin, clofibrate, glyceryl guaiacolate (guaifenesin), and dipyridamole. Drugs that may decrease the anticoagulant effect when given with heparin include *d*-tubocurarine and the quinine derivatives.

MECHANISM OF ACTION

Heparin is a complex anionic mucopolysaccharide with a molecular weight of approximately 12,000. It is stored and probably formed in the mast cells of animal tissues. Heparin inhibits factors involved in the conversion of prothrombin to thrombin. Its anticoagulant effect requires the presence of an alpha globulin known as antithrombin III, the heparin cofactor. Heparin combines with antithrombin III, and in doing so, alters the configuration of that molecule. Antithrombin III is then able to combine with many coagulation proteins and inhibit their activity. Heparin also directly interferes with platelet aggregation.

ABSORPTION AND BIOTRANSFORMATION

Heparin is not well absorbed after oral administration. Subcutaneous, intravenous, and intramuscular routes of administration are effective. Intramuscular injections may cause local or dissecting retroperitoneal hematomas. The drug is metabolized in the liver. A partially degraded form of heparin called uroheparin is excreted in the urine. Heparin *does not* cross the placenta or pass into the mother's milk.

RECOMMENDED READING

Bell, W. R. Hematologic abnormalities in pregnancy. *Med. Clin. North Am.* 61:165–199, 1977.

Courtney, L. D. Amniotic fluid embolism. *Obstet. Gynecol. Surv.* 29:169–177, 1974.

Jaques, L. B. *Anticoagulant Therapy: Pharmacological Principles.* Springfield, Ill.: Charles C Thomas, 1965.

Kakkar, V. V. Deep vein thrombosis, detection and prevention. *Circulation* 51:8–19, 1975.

Kakkar, V. V., Spindler, J., Flute, P. T., Corrigan, T., Fossard, D. P., and Crellin, R. Q. Efficacy of low doses of heparin in prevention of deep vein thrombosis after major surgery. A double blind, randomized trial. *Lancet* 2:101–106, 1972.

Pritchard, J. A. Haematological problems associated with delivery, placental abruption, retained dead fetus, and amniotic fluid embolism. *Clin. Haematol.* 2:563–586, 1973.

(MCM)

Hydralazine (Apresoline®)

INDICATIONS AND RECOMMENDATIONS

Hydralazine is safe to use during pregnancy. It is the drug of choice for the control of moderate to severe hypertension in a patient with preeclampsia-toxemia (PET). This drug may also be used in combination with other agents to control chronic hypertension in obstetric patients.

Significant iatrogenic hypotension can develop when hydralazine is used to treat an acute hypertensive episode in an intravascularly depleted patient with preeclampsia. In order to minimize the chances of this occurring, a 5-mg test dose may be given intravenously 10–15 minutes prior to the administration of more aggressive therapy.

A patient with mild preeclampsia whose fetus still is pulmonically immature may be treated with oral hydralazine in doses of 200 mg/day or less, oral phenobarbital, and bed rest. Failure to maintain diastolic blood pressures below 110 mm Hg on this regimen should prompt the physician to quickly stabilize the patient with intravenous medication and then deliver her of her infant. The renal function of patients with preeclampsia being maintained on oral antihypertensive medication should be monitored daily. Any deterioration of that function should alert the physician to the need for rapid delivery.

Hydralazine alone is a poor choice for the management of patients with chronic hypertension. In order to maximize its long-term effectiveness, it may be necessary to add diuretics and possibly propranolol to the regimen. Since there are objections to the use of these agents during pregnancy, we do not recommend hydralazine as primary therapy for the obstetric patients with chronic hypertension.

SPECIAL CONSIDERATIONS IN PREGNANCY

Acute hypotensive episodes can occur in response to an intravenous bolus of the drug given to a patient with preeclampsia who is intravascularly depleted.

Tachycardia and increased cardiac work and oxygen consumption accompany the intravenous use of hydralazine. This may precipitate angina or myocardial ischemia in a patient with occlusive coronary artery disease. The treatment of symptoms related to increased cardiac work is intravenous propranolol.

Tolerance to the antihypertensive action of hydralazine can develop with chronic administration if a beta-adrenergic blocker (e.g., propranolol) or a diuretic, or both, is not administered. Since there are objections to the use of these agents in pregnancy, methyldopa is a better initial choice for treatment of the pregnant woman with chronic hypertension.

Specific fetal side effects related to hydralazine therapy for the mother have not been described in humans. In animals, however, skeletal defects can be produced that resemble those observed in experimentally induced manganese deficiency states.

Animal experiments have indicated that hydralazine may increase uteroplacental blood flow in sheep with hypertension. There is no convincing evidence in humans that fetal compromise occurs after the administration of this drug in the absence of significant systemic hypotension in the mother.

DOSAGE

Table 7 details how onset, maximal effect, and duration differ with different doses and methods of administration.

ADVERSE EFFECTS

Side effects include palpitations, flushing, nasal congestion, headache, dizziness, anginal attacks, and electrocardiographic changes of myocardial ischemia. Side effects related to chronic

Table 7. Doses of Hydralazine and Methods of Administration

Method of Administration	Dose (mg)	Onset (min)	Maximal Effect (min)	Duration (hours)	Interval (hours)
IV[a]	5–20	10–20	20–40	3–8	3–6
IM	5–20	20–40	40–60	3–8	3–6
Oral	20–50	30–60	90–120	6–8	6–8

[a]The initial intravenous dose should never exceed 20 mg and may be repeated as necessary. The onset of action usually occurs in about 15 minutes. The dose and frequency of administration required for satisfactory blood pressure control are highly variable. After stabilization is achieved, the drug can be administered by a continuous intravenous drip. The daily dose should not exceed 300 mg.

use in doses greater than 200 mg/day include: drug fever, skin eruptions, peripheral neuropathy, blood dyscrasias, mild gastrointestinal symptoms, and an acute rheumatoid state that can progress to the "hydralazine lupus syndrome." Approximately 10%–20% of patients receiving more than 400 mg/day will develop this latter problem.

MECHANISM OF ACTION

Hydralazine reduces vascular resistance by directly relaxing arteriolar smooth muscle. Postcapillary capacitance vessels are much less affected than precapillary resistance vessels. It has been postulated that hydralazine may be able to chelate certain trace metals required for smooth muscle contraction.

Peripheral vasodilatation is not uniform. Vascular resistance in the coronary, cerebral, splanchnic, renal, and uterine circulations decreases more than in skin and muscle. Blood flow in the more dilated circulatory beds usually increases unless the hypotensive effect of the drug is profound.

Hydralazine has no direct action on the heart; homeostatic circulatory reflexes mediated by the autonomic nervous system, however, remain fully functional. Decreased arterial pressure activates baroreceptors to mediate a sympathetic discharge. This results in increased heart rate, stroke volume, and cardiac output. Because this increase in cardiac output partially offsets the effect of arteriolar dilation and limits the hypotensive effectiveness of the drug, when the drug is prescribed for long-term use it is usually combined with a drug that limits the increase in cardiac output.

Renal blood flow and glomerular filtration rates are either unaffected or increased. Hydralazine causes sodium and water retention, with expansion of plasma and extracellular volumes. This is a result of a direct renal mechanism as well as an increase in peripheral plasma renin activity. Increases in renin activity during hydralazine therapy are effectively minimized in the nonpregnant woman by the co-administration of propranolol.

ABSORPTION AND BIOTRANSFORMATION

Hydralazine is fairly completely absorbed after oral administration. Peak serum concentrations are reached 1 to 2 hours after an oral dose. Intravenous administration of a given dose results in higher serum levels than the same dose given orally. About 85% of the circulating drug is bound to albumin.

Acetylation in the liver is the major pathway of biotransformation.

The rate of acetylation is dependent on the genetically determined activity of hepatic N-acetyl-transferase. Therefore, when treated with the same dose of hydralazine "slow acetylators" have higher serum concentrations than "rapid acetylators." In addition, slow acetylators seem to be more prone to develop the hydralazine lupus syndrome.

Very high serum levels may be found in patients with renal insufficiency. Renal excretion of the active drug is not usually an important route of elimination, so uremia probably interferes with biotransformation.

RECOMMENDED READING

AMA Committee on Hypertension. The treatment of malignant hypertension and hypertensive emergencies. *J.A.M.A.* 228:1673–1679.

Koch-Weser, J. Hypertensive emergencies. *N. Engl. J. Med.* 290:211–214, 1974.

Koch-Weser, J. Hydralazine. *N. Engl. J. Med.* 295:320–323, 1976.

Woods, J. R., and Brinkman, C. R., III The treatment of gestational hypertension. *J. Reprod. Med.* 15:195–199, 1975.

(RLB)

Indomethacin (Indocin®)

INDICATIONS AND RECOMMENDATIONS

Indomethacin is relatively contraindicated in pregnancy because other therapeutic agents are preferable. It is used in the treatment of rheumatic and nonrheumatic inflammatory disease, and as an antipyretic agent in Hodgkin's disease when the fever is refractory to other therapy. Indomethacin inhibits prostaglandin synthetase, and its use in pregnancy may theoretically produce premature closure of the ductus arteriosus. Investigators are currently evaluating the usefulness of indomethacin in the treatment of premature labor, but results in large series are not yet published and other agents are available when tocolytic therapy is indicated.

RECOMMENDED READING

Fuchs, A. R., Smitasiri, Y., and Chantharaksri, U. The effect of indomethacin on uterine contractility and luteal regression in pregnant rats at term. *J. Reprod. Fertil.* 48:331–340, 1976.

Goodman, L. S., and Gilman, A. *The Pharmacological Basis of Therapeutics* (5th ed.). New York: Macmillan, 1975. Pp. 341–343.

Roe, R. L. Drug therapy in rheumatic diseases. *Med. Clin. North Am.* 61:405–418, 1977.

(BRS)

Insulin

INDICATIONS AND RECOMMENDATIONS

Insulin is safe to use during pregnancy. It is a naturally occurring polypeptide hormone given parenterally to diabetic patients to lower the blood glucose and correct some of the other metabolic abnormalities related to diabetes. It is the treatment of choice for management of pregnancy in the diabetic. Careful attention to diet is equally important. Frequent blood glucose monitoring is mandatory for any patient taking insulin.

SPECIAL CONSIDERATIONS IN PREGNANCY

Insulin administered exogenously to the mother does not cross the placenta in any appreciable amount. Fetal endogenous insulin, presumably increased due to the effect of maternal hyperglycemia on the fetus, may be responsible for macrosomia and hypoglycemia in the newborn. Fetal hypoglycemia accompanies maternal hypoglycemia. As yet, there is no convincing evidence that there is a detrimental effect of insulin-induced maternal-fetal hypoglycemia on the developing fetus.

DOSAGE

The dose of insulin given to a pregnant diabetic must be individually tailored to that patient's needs. In general, insulin requirements may decrease slightly during the first one-third to one-half of pregnancy, and rapid swings of blood sugar with episodes of hypoglycemia are frequently observed. During the second half of pregnancy insulin requirements often increase to two to three times the prepregnancy dose. There is a tendency toward diabetic ketoacidosis, and hypoglycemia is less common.

Most authorities agree that strict control of blood glucose is most important in managing pregnancy in the diabetic. It is well documented that diabetic ketoacidosis is associated with an extremely high perinatal mortality rate (in some studies as high as 50%). There is some controversy over how low the blood sugar should be maintained. At Yale–New Haven Medical Center and many other centers, the aim is to render the patient "euglycemic," that is, blood sugars should be maintained at levels comparable to those in normal, nondiabetic pregnant women. Fasting plasma glucose is kept in the range of 60–100 mg/dl, and levels 2 hours postbreakfast and in the late afternoon are kept below 120 mg/dl. Although transient hypoglycemia occurs in some patients, it is felt safer to occasionally have to treat this complication (with a high protein snack) than to allow continuous hyperglycemia.

In order to achieve euglycemia during the second half of pregnancy, most long-standing overt diabetics require a mixture of short-acting and intermediate-acting insulin administered twice daily (prior to breakfast and dinner). At Yale–New Haven Medical Center, the starting point usually used is a combination of intermediate and short-acting insulin in a ratio of 2:1 in the morning and 1:1 prior to dinner. The total morning dose is twice the total evening dose. Serum glucose levels are drawn fasting, 2 hours after breakfast, at 4:00 P.M., and at 9:00 P.M. The various components are adjusted with reference to the serum glucose levels obtained at times of maximum and minimum insulin activity.

Many mild diabetics who were on minimal or no insulin prior to pregnancy may be managed with once daily injections of mixtures of short and intermediate-acting insulin in the morning.

The use of low doses of insulin (10 units neutral protamine Hagedorn [NPH] or 20 units NPH with 10 units regular) has been investigated and found to be effective in reducing the incidence of macrosomia in the infants of mild gestational diabetics. These patients would not generally require insulin to maintain euglycemia, but it may be used prophylactically to prevent macrosomia.

ADVERSE EFFECTS

An overdose of insulin can obviously create the side effect of hypoglycemia. Other side effects, not necessarily related to overdosing, include hypertrophy or atrophy of subcutaneous fat at injection sites. Allergic reactions, usually to the beef component, are commonly reported. These often disappear when the patient is switched to pure pork insulin. Circulating antibodies to exogenous insulin are consistently found in treated patients but are rarely a problem.

MECHANISM OF ACTION

Insulin consists of 51 amino acids in the form of a 21–amino-acid "A chain" and a 30–amino-acid "B chain" connected by disulfide linkages. It is produced as a single 84–amino-acid proinsulin chain, but the "C chain" of 33 amino acids (known as connecting peptide) must be cleaved from between the A and B chains in order for the insulin to become metabolically active.

Insulin is necessary for the efficient transport of glucose from blood to tissues other than those of the central nervous system, renal medulla, pancreatic beta cells, and gut epithelium. It also favors hepatic glycogen synthesis and storage of glucose in adipose tissue as triglyceride. Insulin facilitates the transport of ingested amino acids into cells, thus increasing protein synthesis. It inhibits lipolysis and is therefore antiketogenic.

Exogenous insulin can reverse the symptoms of diabetes, i.e., polyuria and polydypsia, by lowering the blood glucose level. It can also reverse diabetic ketoacidosis. It is controversial whether exogenous insulin reverses or slows the vascular complications of diabetes.

Diabetes is characterized as a disease state in which there is a deficiency of insulin that can be either relative or absolute. Many long-standing overt diabetics have virtually undetectable endogenous insulin secretion as measured by C-peptide assay. On the other hand, mild gestational diabetics may have elevated levels of endogenous insulin. In these cases the metabolic abnormality is presumably caused by peripheral resistance to insulin and its increased degradation. This is probably related to the effects of insulinase activity as well as placental steroid and polypeptide hormone production.

ABSORPTION AND BIOTRANSFORMATION

Much controversy exists as to the fate of different forms of insulin in humans. A detailed exploration of this subject is beyond the scope of this book. It is known that insulin is degraded in the liver, kidneys, lungs, and placenta and that some insulin is excreted in the urine. Although some dispute exists, most investigators agree that insulin administered to the mother does not cross the placenta into the fetal circulation.

The duration of action of exogenously administered insulin varies according to the preparation. The insulin is generally derived from pigs (pork insulin), cattle (beef insulin), or is a mixture of the two. The action of purified crystalline zinc insulin (CZI), or "regular," peaks at 1–2 hours and has a duration of 5–6 hours when administered subcutaneously. Semilente insulin, another rapid-acting form, has a peak action similar to CZI, but a longer duration (12–16 hours). An intermediate-acting insulin, neutral protamine Hagedorn (NPH), is a combination of regular insulin and protamine zinc insulin, and has a peak of action at 2–8 hours and a duration of approximately 24 hours. Lente insulin has a similar time course. These peaks and durations of action are related more to absorption than metabolic fate.

RECOMMENDED READING

Coustan, D. R., and Lewis, S. B. Clinical approaches to diabetes in pregnancy. *Contemp. Obstet. Gynecol.* 7:27–36, 1976.

Coustan, D. R., and Lewis, S. B. Insulin therapy for gestational diabetes. *Obstet. Gynecol.* 51:306–310, 1978.

Marble, A., White, P., Bradley, R. F., and Korall, L. P. (Eds.). *Joslin's Diabetes Mellitus* (11th ed.). Philadelphia: Lea & Febiger, 1971.

Pedersen, J. *The Pregnant Diabetic and Her Newborn* (2nd ed.). Baltimore: Williams & Wilkins, 1977.

Skillman, T. G., and Tzagournis, M. *Diabetes Mellitus*. Kalamazoo, Mich.: Upjohn Company, 1973.

(DRC)

Isoproterenol (Isuprel®)

INDICATIONS AND RECOMMENDATIONS

Isoproterenol is used as a cardiac stimulant to raise systemic blood pressure and as a bronchodilator in the treatment of bronchospasm. It is relatively contraindicated during pregnancy because other therapeutic agents are preferable.

Isoproterenol is a pure beta-adrenergic stimulator that increases myocardial strength while relaxing arteriolar and bronchiolar smooth muscle tone. It therefore has positive cardiac inotropic and chronotropic effects in addition to causing peripheral vascular relaxation and bronchodilatation.

Sympathomimetics seem to influence the fetus indirectly by altering uterine blood flow. Uterine vessels only have alpha-adrenergic receptors, and under baseline conditions during pregnancy they are thought to be maximally dilated. Peripheral vasodilation will therefore only shunt blood away from the uterus. This decrease in uterine blood flow may adversely affect the fetus.

RECOMMENDED READING

Goodman, L. S., and Gilman, A. *The Pharmacological Basis of Therapeutics* (5th ed.). New York: Macmillan, 1975. Pp. 493–494.

Smith, N. T., and Corbasciao, A. N. The use and misuse of pressor agents. *Anesthesiology* 33:58–101, 1970.

(MJM)

Isoxsuprine (Vasodilan®)

INDICATIONS AND RECOMMENDATIONS

Isoxsuprine, which is a beta-2 adrenergic agonist, may be administered to pregnant women in order to stop premature labor. A number of such drugs are currently under investigation as tocolytic agents. Only ritodrine has thus far been approved by the Food and Drug Administration for this indication. However, isoxsuprine has been widely used in the United States with significant success, and it has earned a reputation for relative efficacy and safety.

SPECIAL CONSIDERATIONS IN PREGNANCY

Hypotension is the major threat to fetal well-being. This complication is mild, especially when the maternal intravascular volume is adequate. Some recent data suggest an acceleration of maturity of the fetus' pulmonary system when beta-2 agonists are administered to the mother.

A recent retrospective study of outcome for the neonate when the mother was treated with isoxsuprine before giving birth has caused some concern. In this series, 20 babies whose mothers were treated with isoxsuprine and who were delivered of their infants prior to 32 weeks were compared with 20 nontreated controls. In the treated group 7 of the babies died in the neonatal period, as compared with 2 in the control group (not statistically significant). All of the isoxsuprine-exposed babies manifested some degree of hypotension during the first 6 hours of life, as compared to 75% of the babies in the control group ($p < 0.05$). Half of the treated babies developed clinically evident ileus, as opposed to 15% of the untreated babies ($p < 0.05$). These effects on the newborn were most likely to be seen if the interval between the administration of the loading dose of isoxsuprine and the delivery of the baby was short. Neonatal hypoglycemia has also been reported with exposure to beta-2 agonists in utero. Although reports of adverse outcomes in the newborn period are limited in scope and retrospective, they do point out the necessity to be as certain as possible that a woman is truly in premature labor before administering isoxsuprine or any other beta-2 agonist.

DOSAGE

A number of different dosage recommendations have been made. The usual dose is 0.25–0.5 mg/min given intravenously for 8–12 hours. This is followed by intramuscular or oral isoxsuprine at 5–20 mg every 3–6 hours. The intravenous infusion is stopped and considered a failure if labor-like activity persists beyond 1 hour. To prevent hypotension the dose has to be carefully titrated, and the patient should be placed in the left lateral position.

At Yale–New Haven Medical Center a somewhat different dosage schedule has been used over the past 6 years with good results. An initial 20-mg loading dose is given intravenously over 20 minutes with a constant infusion pump. If contractions have not diminished markedly by 40 minutes after the conclusion of the infusion, another 20 mg are administered in the same manner. Once success has been achieved, intramuscular isoxsuprine, 25 mg every 4–6 hours, is given for 48 hours. Then, oral administration is begun at a dose of 50 mg every 6 hours. Although the impression at Yale–New Haven has been that this is a safe and effective protocol, it must be pointed out that premature labor is exceedingly difficult to diagnose. This is borne out by the 60% success rate in some published random prospective studies obtained when dextrose infusion stops "premature labor."

ADVERSE EFFECTS

Because beta-2 receptors are not confined to the uterine muscle but are also responsible for smooth muscle relaxation in arterioles and bronchi as well as being involved in glycogenolysis, the side effects of isoxsuprine may involve any of these systems. Thus, overdosage or rapid infusion may cause hypotension and tachycardia in the mother. Hyperglycemia has also been reported with this drug. The most common side effects are tremor, palpitations, and restlessness. Allergic dermatitis has recently been reported.

Case reports of pulmonary edema occurring in women receiving the combination of a beta-2 agonist and glucocorticoid therapy (in an attempt to enhance the maturity of the pulmonary system in the fetus) suggest that caution be exercised when these classes of agents are combined.

MECHANISM OF ACTION

Isoxsuprine interacts with beta-2 receptors on the myometrial cell membrane to release adenyl cyclase within the cell. This catalyzes the intracellular formation of cyclic adenosine monophosphate which subsequently leads to relaxation of the uterine musculature, presumably through changes in calcium availability.

ABSORPTION AND BIOTRANSFORMATION

Isoxsuprine is largely metabolized by monoamine oxidase. Some is excreted by the kidneys, the rate of excretion being higher in acidic urine.

RECOMMENDED READING

Barden, T. P.   Premature Labor. In *Yearbook of Obstetrics and Gynecology*. Chicago: Year Book, 1977. P. 109.

Brazy, J. E., and Pupkin, M. J.   Effects of maternal isoxsuprine administration on preterm infants. *J. Pediatr.* 94:444–448, 1979.

Casten, O., Gummerus, M., and Saarikoski, S.   Treatment of imminent premature labour. *Acta Obstet. Gynecol. Scand.* 54:95–100, 1975.

Horowitz, J. J., and Creasy, R. K.   Allergic dermatitis associated with administration of isoxsuprine during premature labor. *Am. J. Obstet. Gynecol.* 131:225–226, 1978.

Stubblefield, P. G.   Pulmonary edema occurring after therapy with dexamethasone and terbutaline for premature labor: A case report. *Am. J. Obstet. Gynecol.* 132:341–342, 1978.

(GRD)

Levallorphan (Lorfan®)

INDICATIONS AND RECOMMENDATIONS

Levallorphan is relatively contraindicated in pregnancy because other therapeutic agents are preferable. It is used in the treatment of narcotic-induced respiratory depression. Levallorphan has partial narcotic agonist properties that may increase respiratory depression due to nonnarcotic causes. Such depression may be hazardous to both mother and fetus. Should the use of a narcotic antagonist become necessary, naloxone is the drug of choice.

RECOMMENDED READING

Chang, A., Gilbert, M., Wood, C., and Humphrey, M.   The effects of nalorphine and naloxone on maternal and fetal blood gas and pH. *Med. J. Aust.* 1:263–264, 1976.

Clark, R. B.   Transplacental reversal of meperidine depression in the fetus by naloxone. *J. Arkansas Med. Soc.* 68:128–130, 1971.

Clark, R. B., Beard, A. G., Greifenstein, F. E., and Barclay, D. L.   Naloxone in the parturient patient and her infant. *South. Med. J.* 69:570–575, 1976.

Goodman, L. S., and Gilman, A.   *The Pharmacological Basis of Therapeutics* (5th ed.). New York: Macmillan, 1975. Pp. 271–276.

Nishimura, A., and Tanimura, T.   *Clinical Aspects of the Teratology of Drugs.* New York: American Elsevier, 1976.

(TKM)

Lidocaine (Xylocaine®)

INDICATIONS AND RECOMMENDATIONS

Lidocaine may be administered to pregnant women as an anti-arrhythmic agent. It is used primarily in the emergency treatment of ventricular arrhythmias. Its use as an anesthetic agent will not be considered in this discussion.

SPECIAL CONSIDERATIONS IN PREGNANCY

Lidocaine crosses the placenta, and high blood levels in the mother may be associated with neonatal depression and neurobehavioral changes in the first few days of life. Fortunately, blood levels that are in the therapeutic range for treatment of arrhythmias (2–5 μg/ml) are somewhat lower than the levels found to be associated with these adverse neonatal effects. Very high blood levels in sheep, as well as in experimentally isolated uterine artery segments, may be associated with a transient decrease in uterine blood flow. This has not been reported in humans given lidocaine in therapeutic doses.

DOSAGE

In the emergency management of ventricular arrhythmia, therapy is started with 50–100 mg given intravenously with continuous cardiac monitoring. The rate of administration should be 25–50 mg/min. If the initial dose is not successful, it may be repeated in 5 minutes. Following this, a continuous intravenous infusion may be used (at rates of 1–4 mg/min) to titrate the response.

ADVERSE EFFECTS

Toxic effects of lidocaine occur in the cardiovascular and central nervous systems. Central nervous system effects include light-headedness, drowsiness, tremors, convulsions, and respiratory depression and arrest. Cardiovascular effects include hypotension, cardiovascular collapse, and bradycardia, which may lead to cardiac arrest. These toxic effects are usually seen at serum levels above 5 μg/ml.

MECHANISM OF ACTION

Lidocaine's antiarrhythmic activity is related to a depression in the automaticity of Purkinje cells and a decrease in membrane responsiveness. There is little electrophysiological effect on atrial muscle.

Lidocaine can eliminate premature ventricular contractions and convert a ventricular arrhythmia to normal sinus rhythm. It is not recommended for treatment of supraventricular arrhythmias.

ABSORPTION AND BIOTRANSFORMATION

Lidocaine is not effective when given orally and should be given by the intravenous route. It is primarily metabolized in the liver.

RECOMMENDED READING

Finster, M., Morishima, H. O., Boyes, R. N., and Covino, B. G.   The placental transfer of lidocaine and its uptake by fetal tissues. *Anesthesiology* 36:159–163, 1972.

Goodman, L. S., and Gilman, A.   *The Pharmacological Basis of Therapeutics* (5th ed.). New York: Macmillan, 1975. Pp. 696–697.

Heymann, M. A.   Correlations of fetal circulation and the placental transfer of drugs. *Fed. Proc.* 31:44, 1972.

Mann, L. I., Bailey, C., Carmichael, A., and Duchin, S.   Effect of lidocaine on fetal heart rate and fetal brain metabolism and function. *Am. J. Obstet. Gynecol.* 112:789–795, 1972.

Shnider, S. M., and Levinson, G.   *Anesthesia for Obstetrics.* Baltimore: Williams & Wilkins, 1979. Pp. 28–29, 217, 382.

Teramo, K., Benowitz, N., Hermann, M. A., Kahanpaas, K., Silmes, A., and Rudolph, A. M.   Effects of lidocaine on heart rate, blood pressure, and electrocortigram in fetal sheep. *Am. J. Obstet. Gynecol.* 118:935–949, 1974.

(MJM)

Lithium Carbonate (Eskalith®, Lithane®)

INDICATIONS AND RECOMMENDATIONS

Lithium carbonate may be administered to pregnant women for the treatment of the manic phase of manic-depressive illness. If it is being used for prophylaxis, this drug should be discontinued during the first trimester of pregnancy unless withdrawal would seriously jeopardize the woman or the pregnancy. During pregnancy, the smallest dose possible for acceptable therapeutic effects should be used. This is best accomplished by monitoring plasma lithium levels at least weekly. Frequent small doses should be used to avoid larger fluctuations in maternal plasma concentrations. Individual doses should not exceed 300 mg and should be spaced evenly throughout the day. Major changes in maternal dietary intake or excretion of sodium, especially those causing hyponatremia, should be avoided.

It is advisable to reduce the daily lithium dose by 50% in the last week of gestation and to discontinue it entirely at the onset of labor. Lithium should be reinstituted at prepregnancy dosage immediately after delivery. Since the drug is excreted in the mother's milk and has been associated with toxicity in infants, breastfeeding should be avoided in order to prevent neonatal intoxication.

SPECIAL CONSIDERATIONS IN PREGNANCY

Lithium is not known to have any unusual maternal effects, and the drug is cleared more quickly than it is in the nonpregnant state. Lithium clearance normally ranges from 15–30 ml/min and increases by 50%–100% during the course of pregnancy. This value drops to prepregnancy levels at the time of delivery. Lithium is known to cross the placenta, with concentrations being equal on both sides. It can be teratogenic in rodents if even transiently high lithium concentrations are delivered. Given in divided daily doses and maintained at steady serum concentrations in the human therapeutic range, however, lithium has been found to be without any deleterious effects on either mother or fetus in rodents, rabbits, and monkeys.

A 5-year follow-up study in humans reports that 18 of 166 babies (10.8%) exposed to lithium in utero showed malformations. Thirteen of these involved the cardiovascular system and included ventricular septal defect, coarctation of the aorta, Ebstein's anomaly, mitral and tricuspid atresia, and patent ductus arteriosus. Other malformations reported include anomalies of the central nervous system (aqueductal stenosis with hydrocephalus, spina bifida with meningomyelocele) and external ears. Children exposed to lithium in utero and born without malformation appear to be at no higher risk of developing abnormalities later in life than other children.

Infants born to mothers whose lithium plasma concentrations are in the therapeutic range may exhibit neonatal intoxication. Symptoms associated with neonatal lithium intoxication include cyanosis, lethargy, hypotonia, jaundice, hypothermia, duskiness, poor sucking, poor respiratory effort, low Apgar scores, absent Moro reflex, altered thyroid, and altered cardiac function.

Lithium is secreted in breast milk and has been measured at levels up to half of those found in the mother's serum. Infants breastfed by mothers taking lithium have been reported to be hypotonic, hypothermic, cyanotic, and to have electrocardiographic changes.

DOSAGE

Dose is determined by the severity of the illness and the patient's physical state, body weight, and age. In the treatment of acute mania the usual dosage range is 900–3,000 mg/day with therapeutic serum concentrations in the range of 0.9–1.4 mEq/liter. Plasma concentrations greater than 1.5 mEq/liter produce no clinical advantage and increase the incidence of side effects. As the manic episode subsides, the lithium requirement decreases; the dosage therefore should be decreased fairly rapidly to about 600–1,200 mg/day with plasma levels of 0.7–1.2 mEq/liter. This maintenance dosage must be individually adjusted according to symptoms and side effects.

There is a 4- to 10-day lag period in the onset of therapeutic effect due to the slow rate at which lithium crosses cell boundaries. Should more immediate treatment be required, an antipsychotic agent such as haloperidol or chlorpromazine is generally recommended.

ADVERSE EFFECTS

Initial lithium therapy is associated with a transient increase in the excretion of 17-hydroxycorticosteroids, sodium, potassium, and water. Polydipsia and polyuria frequently occur, and the drug has been implicated in cases of nephrogenic diabetes insipidus. Circulating thyroid hormone levels fall, thyroid ^{131}I uptake is elevated, and plasma protein-bound iodine and free thyroxine levels are reduced. Patients usually remain euthyroid, although some may develop a goiter and become clinically hypothyroid. Reversible electrocardiographic changes can occur. Patients may also develop a fine tremor of the hands.

At toxic levels (2.0 mEq/liter and greater), severe persistent nausea, vomiting and diarrhea, gross hand tremor, slurred speech, muscle twitching, lethargy, seizures, and stupor progressing to coma may appear.

MECHANISM OF ACTION

The precise mechanism of lithium's action is unknown, although it influences nerve excitation, synaptic transmission, and neuronal metabolism in the central nervous system. These effects may be due to altered ion transport or inhibition of adenyl cyclase.

ABSORPTION AND BIOTRANSFORMATION

Lithium is completely absorbed from the gastrointestinal tract within 8 hours, with peak plasma levels occurring in 2–3 hours. It is excreted unchanged, with 95% appearing in the urine, 4%–5% in perspiration, and less than 1% in feces. Approximately 80% of filtered lithium is actively reabsorbed and is competitive with sodium. Sodium depletion will result in a greater reabsorption of lithium and possible toxicity. The plasma half-life in the average adult is 24 hours, with steady state blood levels being reached in 5–6 days.

RECOMMENDED READING

Ananth, J.   Side effects in the neonate from psychotropic agents excreted through breast feeding. *Am. J. Psychiatry* 135:801–805, 1978.

Ayd, F. J.   Hazards to women given lithium during pregnancy and delivery. *Int. Drug. Ther. Newsletter* 8(7):26–27, 1973.

Current Status of Lithium Therapy: Report of the APA Task Force. *Am. J. Psychiatry* 132:997–1001, 1975.

Goodman, L. S., and Gilman, A.   *The Pharmacological Basis of Therapeutics* (5th ed.). New York: Macmillan, 1975. Pp. 791–794.

Schou, M., and Amdisen, A.   Lithium and pregnancy—III. Lithium ingestion by children breast fed by women on lithium treatment. *Br. Med. J.* 2:138, 1973.

Shopsin, B., and Gershon, S.   The current status of lithium in psychiatry. *Am. J. Med. Sci.* 268:307–323, 1974.

Singer, I., and Rotenberg, D.   Mechanisms of lithium action. *N. Engl. J. Med.* 289:254–260, 1973.

Tunnessen, W. W., and Hertz, C. G.   Toxic effects of lithium in newborn infants: A commentary. *J. Pediatr.* 81:804–807, 1972.

Weinstein, M. R., and Goldfield, M. D.   Administration of Lithium During Pregnancy. In *Lithium Research and Therapy*. New York: Academic Press, 1975. Pp. 237–262.

(DJI)

Magnesium Sulfate

INDICATIONS AND RECOMMENDATIONS

Magnesium sulfate is the drug of choice for the prevention of seizures in patients with preeclampsia-toxemia (PET). Women whose toxemia is severe enough to warrant administration of this drug should be delivered of their infants soon after stabilization has been accomplished.

When this drug is given, deep tendon reflexes should be elicited hourly, respirations should be 16/min or more, and urinary output should exceed 30 ml/hr. The administration of magnesium sulfate should be discontinued if deep tendon reflexes are not present or respiratory depression is noted. As diminished urinary output may result in dangerously high serum levels of this drug, in this situation the rate of administration should be altered accordingly. At the Yale–New Haven Medical Center magnesium sulfate is always given by the intravenous route because this permits better control of administration.

The drug should be continued for approximately 24 hours following delivery as prophylaxis against postpartum seizures. If hyperreflexia persists, longer periods of administration may be necessary.

Magnesium sulfate has also been used as a tocolytic agent in attempts to arrest premature labor.

SPECIAL CONSIDERATIONS IN PREGNANCY

Magnesium sulfate may diminish the frequency and intensity of uterine contractions by direct action on the myometrium. In one study comparing the effectiveness of this drug with other agents, magnesium sulfate was successful in arresting premature labor in 77% of cases as opposed to 45% for intravenous ethanol and 44% for dextrose in water.

Magnesium crosses the placenta, and hypotonia, lethargy, weakness, and low Apgar scores have been attributed to fetal hypermagnesemia. Magnesium levels in the cord blood of neonates have been shown to reflect those of their mothers.

DOSAGE

When administered as seizure prophylaxis in PET, magnesium sulfate may be given intravenously or intramuscularly as is shown below:

Intravenous administration via infusion pump
  Loading dose: 4 gm in 250 ml D5/W over 20 minutes
  Maintenance dose: 1–3 gm/hour, titrated by deep tendon reflexes

Intramuscular administration
  Loading dose: 5 gm in 50% solution in each buttock (total, 10 gm) along with 4 gm given intravenously as above
  Maintenance dose: 5 gm in 50% solution every 4 hours after checking deep tendon reflexes, respiratory rates, and urinary output

The intravenous route is always utilized at the Yale–New Haven Medical Center despite claims by some authorities that this is more likely to produce fetal hypermagnesemia. When administered judiciously by a constant infusion and with attention paid to maternal deep tendon reflexes and urine output, this complication has not been observed at our institution. Intramuscular administration, on the other hand, is painful and produces more variable serum concentrations.

When administered in an attempt to arrest premature labor, the drug is given intravenously by infusion pump. An initial 4-gm loading dose delivered over 20 minutes is followed with a continuous infusion at a rate of 2 gm/hour.

Magnesium sulfate toxicity in the mother can be treated by administering 10 gm of calcium gluconate intravenously into a peripheral vein over a 3-minute period.

ADVERSE EFFECTS

Toxic signs and symptoms associated with magnesium sulfate administration do not appear until blood levels exceed 8–10 mEq/liter. At or near this level knee jerks disappear. Between 10 and 12.5 mEq/liter, heart block and peaked T waves on electrocardiogram may be noted, the patient may become obtunded, and respirations may cease. Above this level, cardiac arrest can occur.

MECHANISM OF ACTION

In pharmacological doses magnesium sulfate is a central nervous system (CNS) depressant. It also blocks neuromuscular impulse transmission by diminishing the amplitude of the end plate potential and decreasing its sensitivity to the depolarizing action of acetylcholine. Furthermore, the excitability of muscle fibers to direct stimulation is diminished.

By its action on the CNS and peripheral neuromuscular functions, magnesium sulfate reduces the hyperreflexia associated with PET is an effective prophylaxis against eclamptic seizures. By acting directly on blood vessel walls, this drug causes some vasodilation. This may result in a modest decline in blood pressure and an increase in uterine blood flow in patients with PET.

ABSORPTION AND BIOTRANSFORMATION

When used for the treatment of PET, magnesium sulfate is administered either intravenously or intramuscularly. When given by the latter route, there is a lag of 90–120 minutes before plasma levels reach a plateau. Thirty-five percent of the drug is protein-bound while the rest remains in the ionic form. Magnesium is excreted entirely in the urine, and elevated serum levels may accumulate when standard doses of the drug are given to patients with diminished renal function.

RECOMMENDED READING

Goodman, L. S., and Gilman, A.   *The Pharmacological Basis of Therapeutics* (5th ed.). New York: Macmillan, 1975. P. 722.

Lipsitz, P. J.   The clinical and biochemical effects of excess magnesium in the newborn. *Pediatrics* 47:501–509, 1971.

Lipsitz, P. J., and Inman, C. E.   Hypermagnesemia in the newborn infant. *Pediatrics* 40:856–862, 1967.

Pritchard, J. A.   Standardized treatment of 154 consecutive cases of eclampsia. *Am. J. Obstet. Gynecol.* 123:545–552, 1975.

Pritchard, J., and MacDonald, P.   *Williams Obstetrics* (15th ed.). New York: Appleton-Century-Crofts, 1976.

Wacker, W., and Parisi, A.   Magnesium metabolism. *N. Engl. J. Med.* 278:712–717, 1968.

(PCL)

Mannitol (Osmitrol®)

INDICATIONS AND RECOMMENDATIONS

Mannitol may be administered to critically ill pregnant patients. It is used to promote diuresis and to reduce intracranial pressure. The effect that changes in fetal extracellular fluid volume and intravascular tonicity have on the fetus at various stages of gestation is unknown. For this reason an osmotic diuretic such as mannitol should only be used for life-threatening conditions during pregnancy.

SPECIAL CONSIDERATIONS IN PREGNANCY

The administration of hypertonic solutions to a pregnant woman results in changes in the composition of the maternal extracellular fluid with similar effects on tonicity and blood volume in the fetus. Mannitol crosses the placenta and can result in fetal dehydration. Both of these factors may lead to oxygen and acid-base imbalance in the fetus. In addition, maternal cardiac decompensation could seriously hinder uterine blood flow and thus adversely affect the fetus.

DOSAGE

Mannitol is available for intravenous administration as a 5%, 10%, 15%, 20%, or 25% solution. Specific doses depend upon the underlying disease as well as renal response and fluid balance in a particular patient. Usual adult doses range from 50–200 gm/24 hours. A test dose of 0.2 gm/kg should be given to a patient with marked oliguria or one believed to have inadequate renal function.

ADVERSE EFFECTS

Adverse effects are related to the load of solute administered and the effect of mannitol on fluids and electrolytes. The most serious side effect is cardiac decompensation secondary to circulatory overload. The patient's cardiovascular status, therefore, must be carefully monitored during administration.

MECHANISM OF ACTION

Mannitol is a nonelectrolyte, osmotically active solute that, when excreted by the kidneys, is accompanied by an obligatory osmotic diuresis. The solute prevents reabsorption of water, and urine volume thus can be maintained even in the presence of decreased glomerular function. The concentration of sodium in the tubular fluid is decreased, and the amount of sodium that is reabsorbed is therefore decreased. The excretion of sodium and chloride is increased. In the treatment of elevated intracranial pressure, mannitol again acts osmotically to draw excess fluid across the blood-brain barrier into the intravascular space.

ABSORPTION AND BIOTRANSFORMATION

The drug is poorly absorbed from the gastrointestinal tract and must be administered intravenously. It is confined to the extracellular space, only slightly metabolized, and rapidly excreted in the urine. Approximately 80% of a 100 gm dose appears unchanged in the urine in 3 hours.

RECOMMENDED READING

Goodman, L. S., and Gilman, A. *The Pharmacological Basis of Therapeutics* (5th ed.). New York: Macmillan, 1975. Pp. 819–822.

Pritchard, J. A. Standardized treatment of 154 consecutive cases of eclampsia. *Am. J. Obstet. Gynecol.* 123:543–552, 1975.

Pritchard, J. A., and MacDonald, P. *Williams Obstetrics* (15th ed.). New York: Appleton-Century-Crofts, 1976.

(PCL)

Marijuana

INDICATIONS AND RECOMMENDATIONS

Marijuana is contraindicated during pregnancy. A number of factors are responsible for this recommendation. First, the hazards of cigarette smoking (see *Tobacco*) are, if anything, greater with marijuana, since the smoke is generally inhaled deeply into the lungs and kept there for as long as possible. Second, there is no approved indication for its use, although research into its efficacy as an antiglaucoma agent, an antiemetic, and a tranquilizer is ongoing. Third, Δ^9 tetrahydrocannabinol, the active ingredient of marijuana, is known to cross the placenta, depressing the fetal heart rate and changing fetal electroencephalogram patterns. Finally, indirect data suggest an increased incidence of fetal wastage and congenital anomalies among offspring of marijuana users. Increased numbers of chromosome breaks have been noted in the leukocytes of marijuana users. For the above reasons, it would seem judicious to abstain from marijuana use during pregnancy.

RECOMMENDED READING

Gilmour, D. G., Bloom, A. D., Lele, K. P., Robbins, E. S., and Maximilian, C. Chromosomal aberrations in users of psychoactive drugs. *Arch. Gen. Psychiatry* 24:268–272, 1971.

Goodman, L. S., and Gilman, A. *The Pharmacological Basis of Therapeutics* (5th ed.). New York: Macmillan, 1975. Pp. 306–309.

Mantilla-Plata, B., Clewe, G. L., and Harbison, R. D. Teratogenic and mutagenic studies of Δ^9-tetrahydrocannabinol in mice. *Fed. Proc.* 32:746, 1973.

Montgomery, B. J. High interest in medical uses of marijuana and synthetic analogues. *J.A.M.A.* 240:1469–1470, 1978.

Pace, H. B., Davis, W. M., and Borgen, L. A. Teratogenesis and marijuana. *Ann. N.Y. Acad. Sci.* 191:123–131, 1971.

Stenchener, M. A., Kun, T. J., and Allen, M. A. Chromosome breakage in users of marijuana. *Am. J. Obstet. Gynecol.* 118:106–113, 1974.

(RAC)

Mebendazole (Vermox®)

INDICATIONS AND RECOMMENDATIONS

Mebendazole is contraindicated during pregnancy. It is a broad-spectrum antihelminthic agent effective in the treatment of ascariasis, enterobiasis, trichuriasis, and hookworm disease. It has been found to be embryotoxic and teratogenic at single doses of 10 mg/kg body weight in rats and is therefore not recommended for use during pregnancy.

RECOMMENDED READING

Brugmans, J. P., Thienpont, D. C., vanWijngaarden, I., Vanparijis, D. F., Schuermans, V. L., and Lauwers, H. L.   Mebendazole in enterobiasis. *J.A.M.A.* 217:313–316, 1971.

Drugs for parasitic infections. *Med. Lett. Drugs Ther.* 20:17–24, 1978.

Leah, S. K. K.   Mebendazole in the treatment of helminthiasis. *Can. Med. Assoc. J.* 115:777–779, 1976.

Sargent, R. G., Dotterer, T. D., Savory, A. M., and Lee, P. R.   A clinical evaluation of the efficacy of mebendazole in the treatment of trichuriasis. *South. Med. J.* 68:38–40, 1975.

(TKH)

Meclizine (Antivert®, Bonine®)

INDICATIONS AND RECOMMENDATIONS

Meclizine is probably safe to use during pregnancy. It has been shown to be teratogenic in rodents, but large-scale studies in humans do not show any increase in the rate of severe congenital anomalies when it has been used. It is effective in the prevention of the nausea, vomiting, and dizziness associated with motion sickness, and it may be effective for the relief of vertigo associated with diseases affecting the vestibular system. It is listed in the *Physicians' Desk Reference* as being contraindicated in pregnancy because of the teratogenicity in rodents. Because of the controversy involved, patients should be made aware of this fact before the drug is given.

SPECIAL CONSIDERATIONS IN PREGNANCY

Meclizine crosses the placenta. Large-scale studies in humans show that the rate of severe congenital anomalies in children of mothers who took meclizine during pregnancy is not significantly different from that in the group in which the mothers did not receive antinauseants during pregnancy.

DOSAGE

For prevention of motion sickness, meclizine is given in a dose of 25–50 mg 1 hour prior to departure. It may be repeated every 24 hours as needed for the duration of the journey.

For the control of vertigo it is given 25–100 mg/day in divided doses.

ADVERSE EFFECTS

The most common side effects of meclizine include drowsiness, dry mouth, and, rarely, blurred vision.

MECHANISM OF ACTION

Meclizine is a piperazine antihistamine that depresses labyrinth excitability and vestibular-cerebellar pathway conduction. It inhibits the effects of histamine on capillary permeability and on smooth muscle by competitive inhibition at H_1 receptors. Either stimulation or depression of the central nervous system may occur through an unknown mechanism. It has anticholinergic activity, although no significant effects on the cardiovascular system occur at normal therapeutic doses.

ABSORPTION AND BIOTRANSFORMATION

Meclizine is readily absorbed from the gastrointestinal tract and is widely distributed to body tissues. The exact nature of elimination in man is unknown, but it appears to be extensively metabolized in the liver and excreted in the urine.

RECOMMENDED READING

Biggs, J. S. G.   Vomiting in pregnancy: Causes and management. *Drugs* 9:299–306, 1975.

Goodman, L. S., and Gilman, A.   *The Pharmacological Basis of Therapeutics* (5th ed.). New York: Macmillan, 1975. Pp. 608–611.

Heinonen, O. P., Slone, D., and Shapiro, S.   *Birth Defects and Drugs in Pregnancy*. Littleton, Mass.: Publishing Sciences Group, 1977. Pp. 322–327.

Long, J. W.   *The Essential Guide to Prescription Drugs*. New York: Harper & Row, 1977. Pp. 368–370.

Milkovich, L., and VandenBerg, B. J.   An evaluation of the teratogenicity of certain antinausea drugs. *Am. J. Obstet. Gynecol.* 125:244–248, 1976.

Nishimura, H., and Tanimura, T.   *Clinical Aspects of the Teratogenicity of Drugs*. Amsterdam: Excerpta Medica, 1976.

(DJK)

Meperidine (Demerol®)

INDICATIONS AND RECOMMENDATIONS

Meperidine may be used as an analgesic for pregnant women in labor at term. A narcotic indicated for the relief of moderate to severe pain, it is commonly used in laboring patients, often in combination with a tranquilizer.

It is recommended that if this drug is used in pregnant women, the lowest effective dose should be administered. Infants born to mothers who received meperidine as antepartum analgesia should be observed for respiratory depression. This can be reversed by naloxone. The degree of neonatal respiratory depression produced by any narcotic administered during labor depends on the gestational age and condition of the infant. The magnitude of this effect is inversely proportional to gestational age and may be made greater by birth asphyxia. Meperidine therefore should be used with extreme caution, if at all, during labor that will produce a premature infant.

SPECIAL CONSIDERATIONS IN PREGNANCY

Teratogenicity has not been associated with the use of meperidine during human pregnancies. When given prior to delivery, this drug does not appear to delay labor or to decrease uterine motility. It does not increase the incidence of postpartum hemorrhage, nor does it interfere with postpartum contractions or involution of the uterus.

Administering meperidine to the mother prior to delivery has been associated with neonatal respiratory depression and lower psychophysiological test scores for days after birth. Both of these effects appear to be more marked the longer the drug-to-delivery interval during the 3–4 hours before birth. These are relatively short-term effects and seem to have no long-lasting impact on the infant. It is likely that these effects are related to the presence in the fetus of normeperidine, an active metabolite of meperidine with a longer half-life than the parent compound. In addition, there are individual differences among patients in their ability to metabolize meperidine. If neonatal respiratory depression does occur in a meperidine-exposed newborn, naloxone should be administered immediately to the baby.

As with all narcotic analgesics, infants born to meperidine-addicted mothers are addicted at birth and will experience withdrawal.

Meperidine is secreted into breast milk but in only small amounts. It does not appear to have significant effects on the infant at doses normally prescribed.

DOSAGE

The usual analgesic dose is 50–100 mg IM every 3–4 hours. This dose must be increased if the oral route is used. Intravenous use increases the incidence and severity of untoward effects and subcutaneous administration causes local irritation and tissue induration.

ADVERSE EFFECTS

The most frequently observed side effects seen with meperidine use include light-headedness, nausea, vomiting, dizziness, and sedation. Other, less frequent, side effects include euphoria, dysphoria, dry mouth, flushing, syncope, and palpitations. Meperidine produces less constipation and urinary retention than other narcotic analgesics. Excitation and convulsions may occur at higher doses. Overdosage is characterized by respiratory depression; cold, clammy skin; and extreme somnolence progressing to coma. Death may result from respiratory arrest and cardiovascular failure.

MECHANISM OF ACTION

Meperidine exerts its analgesic effect on the central nervous system. Its exact nature remains unknown, but analgesia is thought to occur through effects on the sensory cortex of the frontal lobes and the diencephalon. In addition, meperidine may interfere with pain conduction or may affect the patient's emotional response to pain.

Meperidine's physiological effects are similar to all of the narcotic analgesics. It produces prompt relief of moderate to severe pain, and the duration of its analgesia is between 2 and 4 hours. Meperidine has little or no antitussive activity in analgesic doses.

ABSORPTION AND BIOTRANSFORMATION

Meperidine is poorly absorbed when given orally; an oral dose is less than half as effective as an identical parenteral dose. Following oral administration, peak analgesia occurs within 1 hour, and its duration is between 2 and 4 hours. After intramuscular injection, peak analgesia occurs within 40–60 minutes and subsides after 2 to 4 hours. Meperidine is primarily metabolized in the liver by hydrolysis and N-demethylation. One metabolite, normeperidine, is active, though less so than meperidine. Five percent of a dose is excreted unchanged.

RECOMMENDED READING

Goodman, L. S., and Gilman, A. *The Pharmacological Basis of Therapeutics* (5th ed.). New York: Macmillan, 1975. Pp. 263–267.

Heinonen, O. P., Slone, D., and Shapiro, S. (Eds.). *Birth Defects and Drugs in Pregnancy*. Littleton, Mass.: Publishing Sciences Group, 1977. Pp. 287–288.

Kuhnert, B. R., Kuhnert, P. M., Tu, A. S. L., Lin, D. C., and Foltz, R. L.

Meperidine and normeperidine levels following meperidine administration during labor: I. Mother. *Am. J. Obstet. Gynecol.* 133:904–908, 1979.

Kuhnert, B. R., Kuhnert, P. M., Tu, A. S. L., and Lin, D. C. Meperidine and normeperidine levels following meperidine administration during labor: II. Fetus and neonate. *Am. J. Obstet. Gynecol.* 133:909–914, 1979.

Morrison, J., Wiser, W. L., Rosser, S. I., Gayden, J. O., Bucovaz, E. T., Whybrew, M. S., and Fish, S. A. Metabolites of meperidine related to fetal depression. *Am. J. Obstet. Gynecol.* 115:1132–1137, 1973.

O'Brien, T. E. Excretion of drugs in human milk. *Am. J. Hosp. Phar.* 31:844–854, 1974.

Petrie, R., Wu, R., Miller, F. C., Sacks, D. A., Sugarman, R., Paul, R. H., and Hon, E. H. The effect of drugs on uterine activity. *Obstet. Gynecol.* 48:431–435, 1976.

(KT)

Mephobarbital (Mebaral®)

INDICATIONS AND RECOMMENDATIONS

Mephobarbital is relatively contraindicated during pregnancy because other therapeutic agents are preferable. This drug is metabolized to phenobarbital. It has properties and uses similar to phenobarbital, but larger doses must be given. Mephobarbital may be prescribed for routine sedation as well as therapy for various forms of epilepsy. If a long-acting barbiturate is necessary during pregnancy, however, phenobarbital is preferable to mephobarbital because it is as effective and much better studied.

RECOMMENDED READING

AMA Drug Evaluations (3rd ed.). Littleton, Mass.: Publishing Sciences Group, 1977.

American Hospital Formulary Service. *Monograph for Mephobarbital.* Washington, D.C.: American Society of Hospital Pharmacists, 1974.

Goodman, L. S., and Gilman, A. *The Pharmacological Basis of Therapeutics.* (5th ed.). New York: Macmillan, 1975. Pp. 210, 220.

(CET)

Metaproterenol (Alupent®, Orciprenaline®)

INDICATIONS AND RECOMMENDATIONS

Metaproterenol may be administered to pregnant patients in aerosol form in the treatment of infrequent, mild episodes of bronchospasm. If the patient remains symptomatic, an oral bronchodilator should be used. Oral metaproterenol may be used as an adjunctive bronchodilator in a pregnant asthmatic who remains symptomatic on maximal doses of theophylline. It should be stated that although no reports of adverse effects have been published thus far, there have not been any large series that have studied the effect of this drug on the human fetus.

The drug must be administered with caution to patients with hyperthyroidism, hypertension, diabetes, congestive heart failure, and coronary artery disease. Furthermore, if it is administered along with another sympathomimetic drug, the potential for adverse side effects may be significantly increased.

SPECIAL CONSIDERATIONS IN PREGNANCY

Metaproterenol has been used to arrest premature labor, although it has not been approved for that use in this country. No unusual maternal effects are reported. No information is available regarding the passage of metaproterenol across the placenta or into breast milk.

In rabbits fetal loss and teratogenic effects have been observed at and above oral doses of 50–100 mg/kg respectively. There are no published reports of teratogenesis in humans using the drug, although no controlled studies are available to establish its safety during pregnancy.

DOSAGE

For oral administration, the dose is 20 mg every 6–8 hours. The onset of action is about 30 minutes. Peak effect occurs in 2 hours and the duration of action is 4–6 hours.

For aerosol administration, the dose is 1–3 puffs (0.65 mg/puff) every 3–4 hours. The onset of action is about 2–10 minutes. Peak effect occurs within 30–90 minutes and the duration of action is 1–5 hours.

ADVERSE EFFECTS

In addition to causing bronchodilation, metaproterenol increases heart rate, stroke volume, and pulse pressure. It also may cause hyperglycemia and an increase in free fatty acids and glycerol. Metaproterenol may also reduce gastrointestinal tone and motility and cause mild general central nervous system stimulation.

Side effects include tachycardia, hypertension, palpitation, nervousness, tremor, nausea, and vomiting. The incidence of side effects is greater when the drug is given orally as opposed to the aerosol route.

MECHANISM OF ACTION

Metaproterenol is a beta-sympathomimetic agonist with predominantly beta-2 activity. It seems to work by stimulating adenyl cyclase, the enzyme that catalyzes the conversion of adenosine triphosphate (ATP) to cyclic adenosine monophosphate (AMP). Cyclic AMP acts locally as a bronchodilator.

ABSORPTION AND BIOTRANSFORMATION

An average of 40% of an oral dose of metaproterenol is absorbed. This is primarily excreted in the urine as glucuronic acid conjugates. Metaproterenol's prolonged duration of action when compared to catecholamine beta sympathomimetic agonists is due to the fact that it is not metabolized by catechol-o-methyl transferase.

RECOMMENDED READING

Drewitt, A. H.   First clinical experience with Alupent—A new bronchodilator. *Br. J. Clin. Pract.* 16:549–551, 1962.

Freedman, B. J., and Hill, G. B.   Comparative study of duration of action and cardiovascular effect of bronchodilator aerosols. *Thorax* 26:46–50, 1970.

Holmes, T. H.   A comparative clinical trial of metaproterenol and isoproterenol as bronchodilator aerosols. *Clin. Pharmacol. Ther.* 9:615–624, 1968.

Hurst, A.   Metaproterenol: A potent and safe bronchodilator. *Ann. Allergy* 31:460–466, 1973.

Rebuck, A. S., and Real, J.   Oral orciprenaline in the treatment of chronic asthma. *Med. J. Aust.* 1:445–446, 1965.

Zilianti, A.   Action of orciprenaline on uterine contractility during labor, maternal cardiovascular system, fetal heart rate and acid-base balance. *Am. J. Obstet. Gynecol.* 109:1073–1079, 1971.

(RJR)

Metaraminol (Aramine®)

INDICATIONS AND RECOMMENDATIONS

Metaraminol, an alpha-adrenergic agent used to increase systemic blood pressure, is relatively contraindicated during pregnancy because other therapeutic agents are preferable. Uterine vessels have only alpha-adrenergic receptors and react to adrenergic stimulus solely by contracting. Such decrease in uterine blood flow may adversely affect the fetus. Should a pressor be needed to treat hypotension in a pregnant woman, ephedrine is the agent of choice.

RECOMMENDED READING

Avery, G. S. *Drug Treatment: Principles and Practice of Clinical Pharmacology and Therapeutics.* Sydney, Australia: Adis Press, 1976.
Goodman, L. S., and Gilman, A. *The Pharmacological Basis of Therapeutics* (5th ed.). New York: Macmillan, 1975. P. 502.
Smith, N. T., and Corbascio, A. The use and misuse of pressor agents. *Anesthesiology* 33:58–101, 1970.

(MJM)

Methenamine Hippurate (Hiprex®, Urex®)

INDICATIONS AND RECOMMENDATIONS

Methenamine hippurate is relatively contraindicated during pregnancy because other therapeutic agents are preferable. It is a urinary tract antiseptic used primarily in the treatment of chronic urinary tract infections. Because the safety of the hippurate salt during pregnancy has not been established, when therapy of chronic urinary tract infections is required and when methenamine is the agent of choice, methenamine mandelate should be administered.

RECOMMENDED READING

Goodman, L. S., and Gilman, A. *The Pharmacological Basis of Therapeutics* (5th ed.). New York: Macmillan, 1975. Pp. 1006–1007.

(GRD)

Methenamine Mandelate (Mandelamine®)

INDICATIONS AND RECOMMENDATIONS

Methenamine mandelate is safe to use during pregnancy. The treatment of choice for urinary tract infections during pregnancy is either a sulfonamide (in the first or second trimester) or ampicillin. Should chronic prophylaxis be required, methenamine mandelate may be used in the pregnant woman. It is most useful in the prophylaxis of *Escherichia coli* cystitis, but it can also usually suppress the common gram-negative offenders, as well as *Staphylococcus aureus* and *Staphylococcus epidermidis* organisms.

SPECIAL CONSIDERATIONS IN PREGNANCY

Methenamine mandelate has been reported to falsely lower the 24-hour urine estriol concentration because formaldehyde destroys estrogen in the urine. The assay is reliable 2 days following discontinuance of the drug.

A study was made of 51 women who received methenamine during pregnancy at a dose of 4 gm daily in divided doses. No difference in fetal outcome was found in this group when compared to controls.

DOSAGE

The recommended dose of methenamine mandelate is 1 gm qid. It is usually given with an acidifying agent, commonly ascorbic acid, 500 mg qid.

ADVERSE EFFECTS

Side effects of methenamine mandelate include nausea and vomiting, and dermatological reactions such as skin rashes, urticaria, and pruritus. Following large doses, bladder irritation, urinary frequency, dysuria, albuminuria, and hematuria may occur.

MECHANISM OF ACTION

Methenamine is decomposed by acids with the liberation of formaldehyde. It is this formaldehyde that is responsible for methenamine's antibacterial effects in the urinary tract. Acidification of the urine is necessary to promote the formaldehyde-dependent antibacterial action. For maximal effectiveness, the urine should be maintained at a pH less than 5.5.

Urea-splitting strains of *Pseudomonas, Aerobacter,* and *Proteus* raise urinary pH and render methenamine inactive unless supplemental urinary acidification is provided. *Candida* infections are resistant to this drug.

ABSORPTION AND BIOTRANSFORMATION

Methenamine is absorbed orally, but 10%–30% decomposes in the gastric juice unless the drug is protected by an enteric coat. The drug is then rapidly excreted in the urine.

RECOMMENDED READING

Goodman, L. S., and Gilman, A. *The Pharmacological Basis of Therapeutics* (5th ed.). New York: Macmillan, 1975. Pp. 1006–1007.

Gordon, S. F. Asymptomatic bacteriuria of pregnancy. *Clin. Med.* 79:22–24, 1972.

(GRD)

Methoxamine (Vasoxyl®)

INDICATIONS AND RECOMMENDATIONS

The use of methoxamine during pregnancy is controversial and, if used at all, it should be restricted to very specific situations. It is an alpha-adrenergic agent used to increase systemic blood pressure. Under baseline conditions during pregnancy, the uterine vessels are thought to be maximally dilated. Alpha-adrenergic stimulation causes vascular contraction and a decrease in uterine blood flow, which may adversely affect the fetus. Methoxamine has been known to produce uterine tetany. Should a pressor be needed during pregnancy, ephedrine is the agent of choice.

RECOMMENDED READING

Avery, G. S. *Drug Treatment: Principles and Practice of Clinical Pharmacology and Therapeutics* (2nd ed.). Sydney, Australia: Adis Press, 1980. P. 1251.
Goodman, L. S., and Gilman, A. *The Pharmacological Basis of Therapeutics* (5th ed.). New York: Macmillan, 1975. Pp. 503–504.
Smith, N. T., and Corbascio, A. The use and misuse of pressor agents. *Anesthesiology* 33:58–101, 1970.

(MJM)

Methyldopa (Aldomet®)

INDICATIONS AND RECOMMENDATIONS

Methyldopa is the drug of choice for pregnant women with mild to moderate chronic hypertension. The action of this drug may be potentiated by the addition of hydralazine or a thiazide diuretic to the treatment regimen. It is recommended that therapy with a thiazide diuretic *not* be initiated during the second half of pregnancy because of its potential for transiently reducing uterine blood flow.

Methyldopa should not be used as primary therapy in a hypertensive crisis.

SPECIAL CONSIDERATIONS IN PREGNANCY

Although methyldopa crosses the placental barrier, it is not known whether the Coombs test can be made positive in the neonates of mothers who take this drug during pregnancy. This neonatal complication seems unlikely because of the duration of therapy necessary before its occurrence in adults. In a series of 117 women given methyldopa during their pregnancies, one mother and none of the neonates developed a positive Coombs test. The same series showed no effect on birthweight and maturity when offspring of patients given the drug were compared to offspring of untreated controls. The authors of this study felt that methyldopa had been demonstrated to be a safe drug for both mother and fetus.

DOSAGE

When given orally, the dose is 250–500 mg every 6–8 hours. The onset of action is 2–4 hours, and the maximum effect is seen in 4–6 hours. The duration of action is 24 hours. At fixed dosage levels, 2–3 days of therapy are required before the full effect of the drug is achieved. After discontinuation of the drug, there is a return to pretreatment blood pressure levels in 24–48 hours.

When given intravenously, the dose is 250–500 mg every 6–12 hours. The onset of action is 2–3 hours. Because of its relatively slow onset of action, this is not the drug of choice for a hypertensive emergency. Given intravenously, this drug may cause enough drowsiness to interfere with the patient's sensorium.

ADVERSE EFFECTS

Methyldopa causes a decrease in peripheral vascular resistance, and postural hypotension may be observed. Cardiac output is reduced by this drug but rarely to a significant degree. Renal and uterine blood flows are maintained in the presence of its hypotensive action.

Side effects include sedation and drowsiness, depression, sodium retention, and nasal stuffiness. A positive Coombs test, which is infrequently associated with a hemolytic anemia, may occur. Positive Coombs tests are said to be present in 20% of patients taking this drug for more than 6 months but are rare prior to that time. Hypertensive crises have been reported when methyldopa has been given in conjunction with propranolol. This is presumably due to a potentiation of the pressor action of alpha-methylnorepinephrine by propranolol.

MECHANISM OF ACTION

Although the exact mechanism of action of methyldopa is unknown, it probably functions as an antihypertensive agent in a variety of ways. It stimulates alpha-adrenergic receptor sites in the central nervous system. It inhibits dopa decarboxylase, which results in a reduction in the production of norepinephrine in postganglionic nerve endings. It is metabolized to alpha-methyl-norepinephrine, which functions as a "false neurohumeral transmitter" at smooth muscle receptor sites. It also suppresses the release of renal renin.

ABSORPTION AND BIOTRANSFORMATION

When methyldopa is administered orally, only 50% or less is absorbed. Methyldopa and its metabolites are weakly bound to plasma proteins. It is metabolized in the gastrointestinal tract and liver and is excreted in the urine largely by glomerular filtration. Unabsorbed drug is eliminated in the feces unchanged. It can be used in patients with impaired renal function but in smaller than usual doses and given at longer than usual intervals.

RECOMMENDED READING

Frohlich, E. D.   The sympathetic depressant antihypertensives. *Drug Ther.* 5:24–33, 1975.

Koch-Weser, J.   Hypertensive emergencies. *N. Engl. J. Med.* 290:211–214, 1974.

Redman, C. W. G., Beilin, L. J., and Bonnar, J.   Treatment of hypertension in pregnancy with methyldopa: Blood pressure control and side effects. *Br. J. Obstet. Gynaecol.* 84:419–426, 1977.

Redman, C. W. G., Beilin, L. J., Bonnar, J., and Ounsted, M. K.   Fetal outcome in trial of antihypertensive treatment in pregnancy. *Lancet* 2:753–756, 1976.

Woods, J. R., and Brinkman, C. R., III   The treatment of gestational hypertension. *J. Reprod. Med.* 15:195–199, 1975.

(RLB)

Methylergonovine Maleate (Methergine®)

INDICATIONS AND RECOMMENDATIONS

The use of methylergonovine maleate is absolutely contraindicated in the pregnant woman. It may be administered postpartum in the management of postpartum uterine atony, hemorrhage, and subinvolution after delivery of the placenta. It should not be given prior to the delivery of the anterior shoulder. It is said to be safer than ergonovine when used in preeclamptic or eclamptic patients since it is associated with fewer pressor effects.

SPECIAL CONSIDERATIONS IN PREGNANCY

Because of its stimulatory effect on uterine muscle—causing tetanic uterine contractions—methylergonovine should not be used at any time during pregnancy, although it may be used post-partum. There are reports that methylergonovine decreases plasma prolactin levels, and controversy exists as to whether or not it has any effect on lactation.

DOSAGE

Oral administration of 0.2 mg every 4 hours × 6 doses is recommended. Intramuscular administration of 0.2 mg after delivery of the anterior shoulder, after delivery of the placenta, or during the puerperium has an onset of action within 2–5 minutes. This dose may be repeated at intervals of 2–4 hours. If essential, methylergonovine may be administered intravenously at a rate not exceeding 0.2 mg/min. Blood pressure should be monitored at all times.

ADVERSE EFFECTS

When given orally, methylergonovine has minimal peripheral vasoconstrictive properties, although it may have a mild pressor effect and cause decreased peripheral blood flow. When given intravenously, however, there may be a significant increase in blood pressure with a subsequent acute hypertensive and cardiovascular crisis. More common adverse reactions include nausea, vomiting, dizziness, headache, tinnitus, diaphoresis, palpitations, and dyspnea.

MECHANISM OF ACTION

Methylergonovine directly stimulates uterine muscle. Peripheral vasoconstriction is also a direct effect. Other complex and sometimes conflicting physiological effects are outside the scope of this discussion.

ABSORPTION AND BIOTRANSFORMATION

The oral tablet is rapidly and adequately absorbed with an onset of action of 5–10 minutes. Methylergonovine is metabolized by the liver and excreted in the feces.

RECOMMENDED READING

Chase, G., et al. (Eds.). *Remington's Pharmaceutical Sciences* (14th ed.). Easton, Pa.: Mack Publishing, 1970. Pp. 952–953.

delPozo, E., Brun de Re, R., and Hinselmann, M. Lack of effect of methylergonovine on postpartum lactation. *Am. J. Obstet. Gynecol.* 123:845–846, 1975.

Goodman, L. S., and Gilman, A. *The Pharmacological Basis of Therapeutics* (5th ed.). New York: Macmillan, 1975. Pp. 540–541, 872–879.

Floss, H., Cassidy, J., and Robbers, J. Influence of ergot alkaloids on pituitary prolactin and prolactin-dependent processes. *J. Pharm. Sci.* 62:699–715, 1973.

(PLR)

Methylphenidate Hydrochloride (Ritalin®)

INDICATIONS AND RECOMMENDATIONS

Methylphenidate hydrochloride may be administered to pregnant women with severe narcolepsy when treatment is considered essential. Although this drug is also used for minimal brain dysfunction in children, as a mild sedative, or as treatment for apathetic or withdrawn senile behavior, narcolepsy, a rare phenomenon, seems to be the only likely indication for its use in the pregnant woman.

SPECIAL CONSIDERATIONS IN PREGNANCY

No information is currently available regarding the effects of this compound on the fetus.

DOSAGE

The usual adult dose is 10 mg two or three times a day. Because of the possibility of degradation in the acid medium of the postprandial gastric fluid, the drug is taken 30–45 minutes before meals. In the treatment of narcolepsy methylphenidate is usually administered prior to important activities.

ADVERSE EFFECTS

Side effects include tachycardia, hypertension, palpitations, anorexia, insomnia, dizziness, headache, dry mouth, and anxiety.

MECHANISM OF ACTION

Methylphenidate is a sympathomimetic central nervous system stimulant. Effects on mental function are somewhat greater than on motor activity. Patients suffering from narcolepsy experience a reduced number of sleep attacks when methylphenidate is combined with changes in daily habits.

ABSORPTION AND BIOTRANSFORMATION

Methylphenidate is deesterified in plasma with less than 1% excreted in urine. The plasma half-life is less than 3 hours.

RECOMMENDED READING

AMA Drug Evaluations (3rd ed.). Littleton, Mass.: Publishing Sciences Group, 1977. Pp. 498–499.
Bioavailability data on Ritalin. Ciba Pharmaceutical Company, Summit, N.J., 1976.
Goodman, L. S., and Gilman, A. *The Pharmacological Basis of Therapeutics* (5th ed.). New York: Macmillan, 1975. P. 365.
Product information on Ritalin. Ciba Pharmaceutical Company, Summit, N.J., 1973.
Safer, D. Depression of growth in hyperactive children on stimulant drugs. *N. Engl. J. Med.* 287:217–220, 1972.

(BDH)

Methysergide Maleate (Sansert®)

INDICATIONS AND RECOMMENDATIONS

Methysergide maleate is contraindicated during pregnancy. It is a semisynthetic derivative of the ergot alkaloids. A theoretical risk of abortion or premature labor exists, and effects of the drug on the fetus are unknown. Effects of methysergide on the mother may be severe.

This drug is effective in the prophylaxis of all types of migraine headaches. It is of no value in treating acute attacks or in the prevention or management of tension headaches. Methysergide has also been of some value in combating intestinal hypermotility in patients with carcinoid and in the postgastrectomy dumping syndrome. Uninterrupted, long-term therapy with methysergide is contraindicated since it may induce fibrotic conditions, including retroperitoneal fibrosis, pleuropulmonary fibrosis, and endocardial fibrosis. Cardiovascular complications include cardiac murmurs; cold, numb, and painful extremities with or without paresthesias; and diminished or absent pulses.

RECOMMENDED READING

AMA Drug Evaluations (3rd ed.). Littleton, Mass.: Publishing Sciences Group, 1977. Pp. 360–361.

Bedard, P., and Bouchard, R.   Dramatic effect of methysergide on myoclonus. *Lancet* 1:738, 1974.

Goodman, L. S., and Gilman, A.   *The Pharmacological Basis of Therapeutics* (5th ed.). New York: Macmillan, 1975. Pp. 540–541, 872–878.

Long, J. W.   *The Essential Guide to Prescription Drugs.* New York: Harper & Row, 1977. Pp. 409–412.

Melmon, K., and Morelli, H.   *Clinical Pharmacology—Basic Principles in Therapeutics.* New York: Macmillan, 1972. Pp. 128–129, 628–629.

Product information on Sansert (methysergide maleate).   Sandoz Pharmaceuticals, East Hanover, N.J., April 12, 1976.

(PLR)

Metronidazole (Flagyl®)

INDICATIONS AND RECOMMENDATIONS

The use of metronidazole during pregnancy is controversial, and, if used at all, it should be restricted to very specific situations. Metronidazole is a broad-spectrum antiprotozoal, antibacterial agent that has been used in treating amebiasis, anaerobic infections (especially *Bacteroides* species), giardiasis, trichomoniasis, vaginitis caused by *Haemophilus vaginalis*, and as a radiosensitizer in the treatment of various tumors. Though metronidazole is probably the single most effective agent available for treating *Trichomonas* infections, the agent is carcinogenic in rodents and mutagenic in bacteria.

In pregnant women metronidazole should not be used when other therapeutic options exist. Clotrimazole vaginal tablets or vaginal cream may offer relief from *Trichomonas* infections, and these agents are preferable during pregnancy.

Since metronidazole is excreted in breast milk, the same precautions should be kept in mind for the nursing mother as for the pregnant woman.

RECOMMENDED READING

Dykers, J. R.   Single-dose metronidazole for trichomonal vaginitis: Patient and consort. *N. Engl. J. Med.* 293:23–24, 1975.

Gyne-lotrimin for vaginal infections. *Med. Lett. Drugs Ther.* 18:66–67, 1976.

Is Flagyl dangerous?   *Med. Lett. Drugs Ther.* 17:53–54, 1975.

Pheifer, T. A., Forsyth, P. S., Durfee, M. A., Pollock, H. M., and Holmes, K. K.   Non-specific vaginitis: Role of *Haemophilus vaginalis* and treatment with metronidazole. *N. Engl. J. Med.* 298:1429–1433, 1978.

Urtasun, R., Band, P., Chapman, J. D., Feldstein, M. L., Mielke, B., and Fryer, C. Radiation and high dose metronidazole in supratentorial glioblastomas. *N. Engl. J. Med.* 294:1364–1367, 1976.

(TKH)

Miconazole (Micatin®, Monistat®, Monistat 7®)

INDICATIONS AND RECOMMENDATIONS

Miconazole may be administered topically to pregnant women for the treatment of candidal vulvovaginitis. It is a broad-spectrum antifungal agent. It should not be used vaginally if membranes are ruptured. An intravenous preparation for the treatment of systemic fungal infections has recently been released. Use of this intravenous agent should be reserved for the treatment of life-threatening fungal infections that are refractory to amphotericin-B.

SPECIAL CONSIDERATIONS IN PREGNANCY

No effects on the fetus directly attributed to miconazole therapy have been reported with the topical use of this drug for the treatment of vulvovaginal candidiasis during pregnancy. No information is available regarding the effects of intravenous miconazole on the fetus. Studies in rats and rabbits have not shown it to be teratogenic; in rabbits, however, high-dose miconazole is associated with an increased percentage of fetal resorptions.

DOSAGE

For the treatment of candidal vulvovaginitis, one applicator dose of the vaginal cream should be inserted high into the vagina at bedtime for 7 days. Recommended doses for intravenous management of systemic fungal infections range from 200–3,600 mg/day for 1–20 weeks, depending on the pathogen.

ADVERSE EFFECTS

Untoward effects of topical miconazole therapy are uncommon and include vaginal burning and itching, pruritus, and cramps. Reported adverse effects of intravenous therapy include phlebitis, thrombocytosis, pruritus, vomiting, and hyperlipidemia.

MECHANISM OF ACTION

Miconazole is effective against pathogenic yeast-like organisms and filamental fungi. It produces relief of the symptoms of vulvovaginal candidiasis. The intravenous form has been effective in the treatment of severe systemic fungal infections.

ABSORPTION AND BIOTRANSFORMATION

Small amounts of miconazole are absorbed from the vaginal mucosa and can be detected in the serum and urine. After intravenous administration, it is rapidly metabolized in the liver, and the inactive metabolites are excreted in the urine.

RECOMMENDED READING

Boelaert, J., Daneels, R., DeMeyere, R., VanLanduyt, H., and Heykants, J. J. P.   Pharmacokinetic profile of miconazole in man. *Eur. J. Pharmacol.* 10:49–54, 1976.

Product monograph on Monistat I.V.   Ortho Pharmaceutical Corporation, Raritan, N.J., 1978.

Sreedhara Sroamg, K. G., Sirsi, M., and Ramananda Rao, G.   Studies on the mechanism of action of miconazole: Effect of miconazole on respiration and cell permeability of *Candida albicans. Antimicrob. Agents Chemother.* 5:420–425, 1974.

(EAC)

Mineral Oil (over-the-counter)

INDICATIONS AND RECOMMENDATIONS

Mineral oil is relatively contraindicated during pregnancy because other therapeutic agents are preferable. This stool softener retards the reabsorption of water from the fecal mass. Because mineral oil may decrease the absorption of vitamin K, leading to a prolonged prothrombin time, sulfosuccinates are preferable as stool softeners in pregnancy.

RECOMMENDED READING

Goodman, L. S., and Gilman, A.   *The Pharmacological Basis of Therapeutics* (5th ed.). New York: Macmillan, 1975. P. 978.

Nelson, M. M., and Forfar, J. O.   Associations between drugs administered during pregnancy and congenital abnormalities of the fetus. *Br. Med. J.* 1:523–527, 1971.

Schenkel, B., and Vorherr, H.   Non-prescription drugs during pregnancy: Potential teratogenic and toxic effects upon embryo and fetus. *J. Reprod. Med.* 12:27–45, 1974.

(RAC)

Morphine

INDICATIONS AND RECOMMENDATIONS

Morphine may be used as an analgesic for patients in early labor at full term. Meperidine is probably a better drug for this purpose, however. There is no solid evidence that morphine can inhibit premature labor or that it offers any advantages in "resting" the patient having a prolonged latent phase.

It is recommended that if this drug is used in pregnant women, the lowest effective dose should be administered. Infants born to mothers who received morphine as antepartum analgesia should be observed for respiratory depression. Should it occur it can be reversed by naloxone. Those infants born to morphine-addicted mothers should be supported through withdrawal during the neonatal period.

The degree of neonatal respiratory depression produced by any narcotic administered during labor depends on the gestational age and condition of the infant. The magnitude of this effect is inversely proportional to gestational age and may be potentiated by birth asphyxia. Morphine, therefore, should be used with extreme caution, if at all, during a labor that will produce a premature infant.

SPECIAL CONSIDERATIONS IN PREGNANCY

Morphine crosses the placental barrier readily. Perfusion experiments conducted on full-term human placentas suggest that morphine has a direct vasoconstrictor action on placental vessels, which may impair the transfer of oxygen and carbon dioxide. Recent data reveal a decreased pH and increased pO_2 in the mother, and decreased pH and base excess in the scalp blood of the fetus when morphine is administered to the ewe. Narcotic agents may cause an accumulation of nonvolatile acids in the fetus; this effect appears to be independent of changes in the mother's blood.

Morphine exerts a direct depressant effect on the respiratory center of the infant. When injected into newborns, it produces a slightly greater respiratory depression than does meperidine. The heightened sensitivity of the newborn is due to an immature blood-brain barrier, which permits a larger amount of administered drug to gain access to the central nervous system. In case of neonatal respiratory depression, a narcotic antagonist should be available. Morphine probably does appear in the breast milk, but no known untoward effects have been reported.

Morphine has been administered in an attempt to arrest premature labor. There is no evidence that it can successfully accomplish this. It has also been recommended as the drug of choice to "rest" a patient who is having a prolonged latent phase of labor. There is no evidence to suggest that this drug has any advantage over several others that could be used for the same purpose.

DOSAGE

Table 8 details how dose and onset and duration of action of morphine differ with different methods of administration.

ADVERSE EFFECTS

Therapeutic doses of morphine depress respiratory rate, minute volume, and tidal volume by means of a direct effect on the brain stem respiratory center. Orthostatic hypotension and syncope may result from peripheral vasodilation due to histamine release. Thus, morphine (and other narcotics) should be used with caution in patients with decreased intravascular volume (e.g., women with preeclampsia) because of the possibility of causing severe hypotension.

Morphine decreases the gastric secretion of hydrochloric acid, as well as pancreatic and biliary secretions. Therapeutic doses cause a marked increase in biliary tract pressure. The constipating effects are due to decreased gastric motility and decreased propulsive contractions in the small and large bowel.

Table 8. Doses of Morphine and Methods of Administration

Method of Administration	Usual Dose (mg)	Onset (min)	Duration (hours)
SC	8–10	15–30	4–5
IM	5–10	10–20	2–4
IV	3–5	3–5	1½–2

Side effects may include nausea, vomiting, dizziness, drowsiness, perspiration, urticaria, and respiratory depression. Allergic phenomena may also occur.

MECHANISM OF ACTION

The analgesic effects of morphine are due to its action on the central nervous system. There is no effect on peripheral nerves. Morphine produces analgesia, drowsiness, changes in mood, and mental clouding. Continuous dull pain is relieved more effectively than sharp intermittent pain.

ABSORPTION AND BIOTRANSFORMATION

Morphine is relatively ineffective orally but may be administered by subcutaneous, intramuscular, or intravenous routes. The major detoxification pathway is conjugation with glucuronic acid.

Some phenothiazines reduce the amount of narcotic required to produce a given level of analgesia. Unfortunately, the respiratory depressant effect may be enhanced, and the hypotensive effects of the phenothiazine become an additional complication.

RECOMMENDED READING

Chang, A., Wood, C., Humphrey, M., Gilbert, M., and Wagstaff, C. The effect of narcotics on fetal acid base status. *Br. J. Obstet. Gynaecol.* 83:56–61, 1976.

Goodman, L. S., and Gilman, A. *The Pharmacological Basis of Therapeutics* (5th ed.). New York: Macmillan, 1975. Pp. 245–283.

Petrie, R., Wu, R., Miller, F. C., Sacks, D. A., Sugarman, R., Paul, R. H., and Hon, E. H. The effect of drugs on uterine activity. *Obstet. Gynecol.* 48:431–435, 1976.

(KT)

Nalorphine (Nalline®)

INDICATIONS AND RECOMMENDATIONS

Nalorphine is relatively contraindicated during pregnancy because other therapeutic agents are preferable. It has been used for treatment of narcotic-induced respiratory depression. Nalorphine has partial agonist properties that may increase respiratory depression due to nonnarcotic causes, and such depression may be hazardous to both mother and fetus. Should the use of a narcotic antagonist become necessary, naloxone is the drug of choice.

RECOMMENDED READING

Chang, A., Gilbert, M., Wood, C., and Humphrey, M. The effects of nalorphine and naloxone on maternal and fetal blood gas and pH. *Med. J. Aust.* 1:263–264, 1976.

Clark, R. B. Transplacental reversal of meperidine depression in the fetus by naloxone. *J. Arkansas Med. Soc.* 68:128–130, 1971.

Clark, R. B., Beard, A. G., Greifenstein, F. E., and Barclay, D. L. Naloxone in the parturient patient and her infant. *South. Med. J.* 69:570–575, 1976.

Goodman, L. S., and Gilman. A. *The Pharmacological Basis of Therapeutics* (5th ed.). New York: Macmillan, 1975. Pp. 271–276.

Nishimura, A., and Tanimura, T. *Clinical Aspects of the Teratology of Drugs.* New York: American Elsevier, 1976.

(TKM)

Naloxone (Narcan®)

INDICATIONS AND RECOMMENDATIONS

Naloxone is safe to use during pregnancy. It is the drug of choice for the treatment of narcotic-induced respiratory depression in mother or neonate, or both. Naloxone may be administered immediately after birth to the depressed neonate whose mother has been treated with a narcotic analgesic. Alternatively, a dose given to the mother 10 to 15 minutes before delivery of the infant will decrease neonatal respiratory depression secondary to maternal narcotic administration.

Naloxone is also used in the diagnosis of narcotic addiction. It would probably be inappropriate to use it for this purpose in the pregnant woman as the sudden withdrawal might be deleterious to the fetus.

SPECIAL CONSIDERATIONS IN PREGNANCY

Animal studies have not shown any teratogenic effects. It does cross the placenta and can reverse neonatal depression secondary to narcotic administration to the mother.

DOSAGE

The intravenous route of administration produces the most rapid effect. Repeat doses may be required at 1–2-hour intervals, depending on the specific agent that is causing the depression. Supplemental intramuscular doses have a longer lasting effect. For adults the dose is 0.4 mg given IV, IM, or SC, repeated at

2–3-minute intervals × 2 if there is no immediate effect. For the neonate the dose is 0.01 mg/kg given IV, IM, or SC.

ADVERSE EFFECTS

In opiate-dependent subjects, naloxone produces a moderate to severe withdrawal syndrome that appears within minutes and lasts approximately 2 hours. Naloxone itself is devoid of narcotic agonist properties, and doses of up to 12 mg produce no discernible effect in the absence of a narcotic.

MECHANISM OF ACTION

Naloxone displaces morphine-like drugs from their specific receptor sites. It reverses narcotic-induced respiratory depression, analgesia, sedation, hypotension, and pupillary constriction. It also reverses the depressant effects of narcotic antagonists and congeners including nalorphine, levallorphan, pentazocine, and diphenoxylate.

ABSORPTION AND BIOTRANSFORMATION

Naloxone is metabolized in the liver primarily by glucuronidation.

RECOMMENDED READING

Chang, A., Gilbert, M., Wood, C., and Humphrey, M.   The effects of nalorphine and naloxone on maternal and fetal blood gas and pH. *Med. J. Aust.* 1:263–264, 1976.

Clark, R. B.   Transplacental reversal of meperidine depression in the fetus by naloxone. *J. Arkansas Med. Soc.* 68:128–130, 1971.

Clark, R. B., Beard, A. G., Greifenstein, F. E., and Barclay, D. L.   Naloxone in the parturient patient and her infant. *South. Med. J.* 69:570–575, 1976.

Goodman, L. S., and Gilman, A.   *The Pharmacological Basis of Therapeutics* (5th ed.). New York: Macmillan, 1975. Pp. 271–276.

Nishimura, A., and Tanimura, T.   *Clinical Aspects of the Teratology of Drugs.* New York: American Elsevier, 1976.

(TKM)

Nitrites: Amyl nitrite, Erythrityl tetranitrate (Cardilate®), Isosorbide dinitrate (Isordil®, Sorbitrate®), Nitroglycerine (Nitro-Bid®, Nitrol®, Nitrostat®), Pentaerythritol tetranitrate (Peritrate®)

INDICATIONS AND RECOMMENDATIONS

Nitrites may be administered to pregnant women with angina pectoris. In such patients, however, it would be best to treat the condition with bedrest rather than with these drugs. If, however, nitrites must be used, they should be given in the lowest effective dose and for treatment of acute attacks only. Fortunately, angina pectoris is not a disease frequently encountered in women of childbearing age.

SPECIAL CONSIDERATIONS IN PREGNANCY

There are no data concerning the ability of these compounds to cross the placental barrier. It may be assumed, however, that fetal and maternal blood levels of nitroglycerine equilibrate and that physiological effects on the fetus are similar to those on its mother. There are no reports available on effects on the fetus due to maternal ingestion of these drugs.

DOSAGE

Table 9 details dose, method of administration, and onset and duration of action of the nitrites. These drugs are used as needed for angina pectoris, and in the average patient would not be used daily.

ADVERSE EFFECTS

The most common side effects of these compounds are headache, dizziness, weakness, postural hypotension, and a typical flush on the head, neck, and clavicular area. In very high doses, the nitrite ion can significantly oxidize hemoglobin to methemoglobin.

MECHANISM OF ACTION

These drugs are thought to act through nitrite receptors to nonspecifically relax smooth muscle. They are functional an-

Table 9. Dose, Onset and Duration of the Nitrites

Drug	Method of Administration	Onset	Duration
Amyl nitrite	Inhale 0.18–0.3 ml	30 sec	3–5 min
Nitroglycerin	0.15–0.6 mg sublingual	3 min	9–11 min
Nitroglycerin ointment	2% topical to skin	30–60 min	3 hours
Erythrityl tetranitrate	15–60 mg PO per dose	30 min	4 hours
	5–15 mg sublingual	5 min	4 hours
Pentaerythritol tetranitrate	10–40 mg PO per dose	30 min	4–5 hours
Isosorbide dinitrate	10–60 mg PO per dose	15–30 min	4–6 hours
	2.5–10 mg sublingual	2–5 min	1–2 hours

tagonists of norepinephrine, acetylcholine, and histamine and do not prevent cells from responding to appropriate stimuli.

Their predominant therapeutic actions are on vascular smooth muscle. Generalized vasodilation occurs, but venous dilation is a prominent factor in the blood pressure response to nitroglycerin. Blood pressure is decreased secondarily to generalized vasodilation; but, since the sympathetic nervous system is not blocked, tachycardia may occur. The extent of the hypotension depends on the patient's position. In people with angina, venous dilation presumably causes peripheral pooling of blood, with a decrease in cardiac output and work load.

The nitrites are effective in the treatment of acute attacks of angina. They also can prevent these attacks when taken shortly before periods of stress. The studies on the long-acting nitrites used for chronic prophylaxis of angina are difficult to assess. They may be no better than placebos.

ABSORPTION AND BIOTRANSFORMATION

Most organic nitrites (nitroglycerin and the long-acting compounds) are readily absorbed from the sublingual mucosa. When administered by this route, their effects are more intense and predictable than when they are administered orally. Degradation of these compounds takes place rapidly in the liver, so that even though they are well absorbed from the gastrointestinal tract, little drug reaches the systemic circulation in active form. Sustained-release oral preparations have been formulated and may deliver enough drug to provide a prolongation in action. Nitroglycerine and other organic nitrates are also absorbed through the skin. These compounds are rapidly dinitrated in the liver, and metabolites are excreted in the urine.

RECOMMENDED READING

American Hospital Formulary Service. *Monograph for Nitrostat.* Washington, D.C.: American Society of Hospital Pharmacists, 1975.
Goodman, L. S., and Gilman, A. *The Pharmacological Basis of Therapeutics* (5th ed.). New York: Macmillan, 1975. Pp. 727–735.

(DJK)

Nitrofurantoin (Furadantin®, Macrodantin®)

INDICATIONS AND RECOMMENDATIONS

Nitrofurantoin may be administered to pregnant patients in treatment of asymptomatic or symptomatic bacteriuria caused by sensitive organisms. It is an antimicrobial used in the treatment of acute uncomplicated lower urinary tract infections as well as for long-term suppression in patients with chronic bacteriuria. It is effective against *Escherichia coli,* enterococcus, and staphylococcus, but ineffective against *Pseudomonas, Proteus,* or *Klebsiella.* It should not be used in patients with compromised renal function, including those with hypertensive, toxemic, or diabetic nephropathy.

SPECIAL CONSIDERATIONS IN PREGNANCY

There are no unique maternal problems if nitrofurantoin is taken during pregnancy. Hemolytic anemia has been reported in newborns of mothers taking this drug prior to delivery. This problem is evidently related to immaturity of red cell membrane enzyme systems, and for this reason, it is best to prescribe another antibiotic during the third trimester of pregnancy.

DOSAGE

The dose of nitrofurantoin for treatment of acute urinary tract infections is 50–100 mg by mouth qid. The dose used for long-term suppressive therapy is 50–100 mg by mouth qhs.

ADVERSE EFFECTS

Side effects of nitrofurantoin include nausea and vomiting, and teeth discoloration in young children. The most serious side effect is peripheral neuritis, which is usually seen in patients with renal failure. This complication may be fatal, and its most common manifestation is an ascending motor and sensory polyneuropathy. The drug should be stopped in patients who complain of paresthesias and other early signs of neuritis. Pulmonary reactions have been observed in patients on long-term therapy, although acute reactions may occur within the first week of therapy. Hemolytic anemia may be seen in patients with glucose 6-phosphate dehydrogenase (G6PD) deficiency. Hepatotoxicity has also been reported.

MECHANISM OF ACTION

Nitrofurantoin interferes with early stages of bacterial carbohydrate metabolism by inhibiting acetyl-coenzyme A activity. It is bacteriostatic in vivo.

ABSORPTION AND BIOTRANSFORMATION

Nitrofurantoin is absorbed from the gastrointestinal tract. The macrocrystal form (Macrodantin®) seems to be absorbed more slowly than the usual form and is said to be associated with less gastrointestinal intolerance. Despite good absorption, therapeutically effective serum levels are not reached with the usual oral dose. The serum half-life is only 20 minutes because of rapid tissue breakdown and urinary excretion. One-third of an oral dose appears in an active form in the urine. Uremic patients excrete very little nitrofurantoin in the urine, making the drug useless in such patients.

RECOMMENDED READING

Crawan, R. S.   Furadantin neuropathy. *Aust. N.Z. J. Med.* 1:246–249, 1971.
Kalowski, S., Radford, N., and Kincaid-Smith, P.   Crystalline and macrocrystalline nitrofurantoin in the treatment of urinary tract infection. *N. Engl. J. Med.* 290:385–387, 1974.
Urinary antiseptics (Today's Drugs).   *Br. Med. J.* 2:812–814, 1968.

(GRD)

Norepinephrine (Levophed®)

INDICATIONS AND RECOMMENDATIONS

The use of norepinephrine in pregnancy is controversial and if used at all, it should be restricted to life-threatening situations. It is an adrenergic agent that has a preponderance of alpha activity and is used to treat hypotension. An increased frequency of uterine contractions has been noticed with its use. In addition, the uterine vasculature, thought to be maximally dilated during pregnancy, reacts to adrenergic stimulus solely by contraction. Such a decrease in uterine blood flow may adversely affect the fetus. Should an adrenergic agent be required to treat hypotension during pregnancy, ephedrine is the drug of choice.

RECOMMENDED READING

Avery, G. S.   *Drug Treatment: Principles and Practice of Clinical Pharmacology and Therapeutics* (2nd ed.). Sydney, Australia: Adis Press, 1980. P. 91.
Goodman, L. S., and Gilman, A.   *The Pharmacological Basis of Therapeutics* (5th ed.). New York: Macmillan, 1975. Pp. 491–493.
Smith, N. T., and Corbascio, A.   The use and misuse of pressor agents. *Anesthesiology* 33:58–101, 1970

(MJM)

Nystatin (Mycostatin®, Nilstat®)

INDICATIONS AND RECOMMENDATIONS

Nystatin is safe to use during pregnancy for the treatment of *Candida* infections of the skin, mucous membranes, and intestinal tract. It should not be applied vaginally when membranes have ruptured.

SPECIAL CONSIDERATIONS IN PREGNANCY

Since nystatin is effectively contained at the site of application, it is safe to use during pregnancy. Its use has not been associated with teratogenesis.

DOSAGE

Oral (for intestinal fungal infections)
   500,000–1,000,000 units tid for 48 hours after clinical cure

Oral (for thrush)
   400,000–600,000 units qid; retain in mouth as long as possible

Topical (for cutaneous or mucocutaneous candidiasis)
   Apply liberally bid; continue application for 1 week after clinical cure

Vaginal (for vulvovaginal candidiasis)
   100,000–200,000 units via applicator placed daily high in the vagina

ADVERSE EFFECTS

Untoward effects of nystatin are uncommon. Mild nausea and vomiting may occur after oral administration.

MECHANISM OF ACTION

Nystatin is bound to fungal cell membranes, creating a change in permeability of the membrane. This change allows leakage of essential small molecules out of the cell.

ABSORPTION AND BIOTRANSFORMATION

Nystatin is not absorbed from the skin or mucous membranes. Absorption from the gastrointestinal tract is negligible and results in no detectable blood levels at recommended doses.

RECOMMENDED READING

Burrow, G. N., and Ferris, T. F. *Medical Complications During Pregnancy.* Philadelphia: Saunders, 1975. Pp. 470–471.
Goodman, L. S., and Gilman, A. *The Pharmacological Basis of Therapeutics* (5th ed.). New York: Macmillan, 1975. Pp. 1235–1236.

(TKM)

Paraldehyde (Paral®)

INDICATIONS AND RECOMMENDATIONS

Paraldehyde is relatively contraindicated during pregnancy because other therapeutic agents are preferable. It is a short-acting sedative-hypnotic used in the treatment of abstinence (from alcohol) phenomena and other psychiatric states characterized by excitement. It has also been used in the emergency treatment of various types of seizures.

Because of numerous reports of death from paraldehyde intoxication, and because of the tendency of the drug to become contaminated by corrosive decomposition products, it has been replaced by other drugs in most situations. Paraldehyde readily crosses the placenta and depression of the fetus has been reported with its use. It is recommended that agents such as magnesium sulfate, used for the prevention of convulsions in preeclampsia, and phenothiazine drugs, used as psychotherapeutic agents, be administered instead of paraldehyde.

RECOMMENDED READING

American Hospital Formulary Service. *Monograph on Paraldehyde.* Section 28:24, Washington, D.C.: American Society of Hospital Pharmacists, July, 1975.

Goodman, L. S., and Gilman, A. *The Pharmacological Basis of Therapeutics* (5th ed.). New York: Macmillan, 1975. Pp. 131–132.

Kittel, J. Paraldehyde toxicity. *Hosp. Pharmacy* 8:8, 1973.

(CET)

Pargyline (Eutonyl®)

INDICATIONS AND RECOMMENDATIONS

Pargyline is contraindicated during pregnancy. It is a monoamine oxidase inhibitor that has been used as an antihypertensive agent and also has antidepressive properties.

Inhibition of monamine oxidase in postganglionic nerve endings results in the accumulation of dopamine and octopamine at these sites. These substances act either as false neurohumeral transmitters or permit a negative feedback inhibition of tyrosine hydroxylase. The latter is an integral part of norepinephrine biosynthesis.

This drug may precipitate a severe hypertensive crisis when a patient eats food that is rich in tyramine while the drug is being ingested. A hypertensive crisis can also occur when pargyline is prescribed concurrently with amphetamine, ephedrine, imipramine, phenylephrine, metaraminol, and phenylpropanolamine.

Because other agents are more effective and less dangerous, pargyline has no role in the management of hypertension in the pregnant woman.

RECOMMENDED READING

Frohlich, E. D. The sympathetic depressant anti-hypertensives. *Drug Ther.* 5:24–33, 1975.

Goodman, L. S., and Gilman, A. *The Pharmacological Basis of Therapeutics* (5th ed.). New York: Macmillan, 1975. Pp. 715–716.

Levin, N. W., Kravitz, A., Navarro, O. M., and Ritzlin, P. Anti-hypertensive therapy. *Hosp. Formu. Manag.* 6:9–15, 1971.

(RLB)

Penicillins: Amoxicillin (Polymox®), Ampicillin (Penbritin®), Carbenicillin (Geopen®), Cloxacillin (Tegopen®), Dicloxacillin (Veracillin®), Methicillin (Staphcillin®), Nafcillin (Unipen®), Oxacillin (Prostaphlin®), Penicillin G, Penicillin V

INDICATIONS AND RECOMMENDATIONS

Penicillins are safe to use during pregnancy in nonallergic patients. These compounds are among the most effective and least toxic antimicrobials available. The family consists of natural and semisynthetic compounds that have individual spectra and pharmacological properties.

SPECIAL CONSIDERATIONS IN PREGNANCY

The use of ampicillin can lower urine estriols, presumably by destroying gastrointestinal flora and interfering with enterohepatic recirculation of estrogens. Estriol values return to normal 2 days after the drug is discontinued. Although penicillin and its derivatives appear in the amniotic fluid and fetal blood and tissues, these drugs do not appear to be teratogenic. Penicillin does appear in breast milk and may cause diarrhea and candidiasis in the nursing infant.

DOSAGE

Table 10 details recommended dosages of the penicillins.

Table 10. Dosage Chart for Penicillins

Drug	Oral Dosage	Oral Interval (hours)	Parenteral Dosage	Parenteral Interval (hours)	Usual Maximum Dose/Day	Dosage Interval for Creatinine Clearance (ml/min) 80–50	50–10	Less than 10
Amoxicillin	750–1,500 mg/day	q8			3 gm	8 hours	12 hours	16 hours
Ampicillin[a]	2–4 gm/day	q6	2–12 gm/day	q6	12 gm	8 hours	8 hours	12 hours
Carbenicillin	4–8 tabs/day[b]	q6	30–40 gm/day[c]	q6	40 gm	6 hours	2–4 gm q6h[d]	2 gm q12h
Cloxacillin	2–4 gm/day	q6			4 gm	8 hours	8 hours	12 hours
Dicloxacillin	1–2 gm/day	q6			4 gm	8 hours	8 hours	12 hours
Methicillin			4–12 gm/day	q4–6	12 gm	6 hours	8 hours	12 hours
Nafcillin	2–4 gm/day	q6	2–12 gm/day	q4–6	12 gm	6 hours	8 hours	12 hours
Penicillin G	1.6–3.2 MU/day	q6	1.2–24 MU/day	q4–12[e]	24 MU/day	(no change)	(change not required)[f]	12 hours
Penicillin V	1.6–3.2 MU/day[g]	q6			6.4 MU/day	8 hours	8 hours	12 hours
Oxacillin	2–4 gm/day	q6	2–12 gm/day	q4–6	12 gm	8 hours	8 hours	12 hours

a In meningitis, dose should be given q4h. Ampicillin has been associated with a falsely low 24-hour urine estriol during pregnancy.
b Tablets contain 382 mg of indanyl sodium carbenicillin.
c To be given for septicemia or other severe infections; 4–8 gm/day is usually sufficient for urinary tract infections.
d Parenteral dose for adults.
e Intervals of 12 hours between doses for penicillin G procaine only.
f Patients with severe renal insufficiency should be given no more than one-third to one-half the maximum daily dosage, i.e., instead of giving 24 MU per day, 10 MU should be given. Patients on lower doses usually tolerate full dosage even with severe renal insufficiency.
g 1 gm is equal to 1,600 units.
NOTE: MU = million units.

ADVERSE EFFECTS

The penicillins are reported to be among the most common causes of drug allergy. The severity of allergic reactions ranges from a mild rash to anaphylaxis. Interstitial nephritis has been associated primarily with methicillin while oxacillin has been implicated as the cause of a reversible hepatotoxicity and neutropenia. The most frequent side effects of orally administered penicillins are nausea, vomiting, epigastric distress, diarrhea, and black hairy tongue. Penicillins are irritating to the central and peripheral nervous systems, especially at very high doses and in patients with impaired renal function. As parenteral formulations may contain large quantities of sodium or potassium, electrolyte imbalances may occur with intravenous therapy. Candidal vaginitis is a common sequel to penicillin therapy, presumably because of suppression of normal vaginal flora.

MECHANISM OF ACTION

This group of antibiotics acts by interfering with cell wall synthesis. They are therefore more effective when organisms are actively dividing.

In general, the penicillins are active against gram-positive cocci and bacilli and some gram-negative bacilli; some have a broader spectrum and are active against many gram-negative bacilli. None of the penicillins are active against viruses, mycobacteria, plasmodia, fungi, or rickettsiae.

ABSORPTION AND BIOTRANSFORMATION

The penicillins are variably absorbed from the gastrointestinal tract and are widely distributed throughout the body. They diffuse into ascitic fluid and attain high concentrations in lungs, intestine, and liver. The penicillins are concentrated in bile; only small amounts diffuse into cerebrospinal fluid, with penetration being greater through inflamed meninges. Penicillins are bound to plasma proteins to varying degrees; the free drug appears to be the active form. Most penicillins are primarily excreted unchanged in the urine, with only small amounts being inactivated by the liver or excreted in bile. The latter two modes of elimination assume more importance in the presence of renal failure. The half-lives of the penicillins are in general short, ranging from 30–90 minutes. In an anuric patient, half-lives may be as high as 10 hours. Concomitant administration of probenecid increases and prolongs serum penicillin levels by competitively inhibiting renal tubular secretion and thus slowing the rate of penicillin elimination.

RECOMMENDED READING

Anderson, G. G., Hobbins, J. C., and Speroff, L.   Obstetrical Management of the High Risk Patient. In G. Burrow and T. F. Ferris (Eds.), *Medical Complications of Pregnancy*. Philadelphia: Saunders, 1975. P. 910.

Handbook of Antimicrobial Therapy. The Medical Letter on Drugs and Therapeutics (Rev. ed.). New Rochelle, N.Y.: The Medical Letter, 1978.

Philipson, A.   Pharmacokinetics of ampicillin during pregnancy. *J. Infec. Dis.* 136:370–376, 1977.

(GRD)

Phenacetin

INDICATIONS AND RECOMMENDATIONS

Phenacetin is generally not available as a single drug. It is always used in combination with acetylsalicylic acid, salicylamide, caffeine, and so on. Because of concern about the antiplatelet activity of aspirin, phenacetin in combination with aspirin-like compounds is not recommended for use during pregnancy.

RECOMMENDED READING

Goodman, L. S., and Gilman, A.   *The Pharmacological Basis of Therapeutics* (5th ed.). New York: Macmillan, 1975. Pp. 343–348.

(RAC)

Phenmetrazine (Preludin®)

INDICATIONS AND RECOMMENDATIONS

Phenmetrazine is contraindicated during pregnancy. It is used as a short-term (4–6 weeks) adjunct to a weight reduction program for obese patients. The anorexic effect of phenmetrazine is temporary and believed to be mediated through direct stimulation of the hypothalamic satiety center. Side effects that can occur in the mother include palpitations, elevation of blood pressure, and tachycardia. Cases of skeletal and visceral anomalies in infants whose mothers have taken phenmetrazine during pregnancy have been reported, but no causal relationship can be proved. Studies performed in pups during weaning, whose mothers were given phenmetrazine in pregnancy, demonstrated a decrease in survival and growth rate. Since it is not appropriate for pregnant women to participate in weight reduction programs, phenmetrazine has no role during pregnancy.

RECOMMENDED READING

Cahen, M. L. Evaluation of the teratogenicity of drugs. *Clin. Pharmacol. Ther.* 5:480–514, 1964.

Craddock, D. Anorectic drugs: Use in general practice. *Drugs* 11:378–393, 1976.

Product information on Preludin. Boehringer Ingelheim Ltd., Ridgefield, Conn., May, 1976.

(BDH)

Phenobarbital

INDICATIONS AND RECOMMENDATIONS

Phenobarbital may be administered to pregnant women in the treatment of grand mal and focal seizures and may be administered as a sedative to patients with mild to moderate preeclampsia. It is not recommended for the stimulation of fetal hepatic enzymes. Phenobarbital may be given to breastfeeding mothers, but drowsiness should be looked for in the nursing infant.

The following recommendations have been made in a bulletin published in 1979 by the American Academy of Pediatrics Committee on Drugs in collaboration with the American College of Obstetrics and Gynecology (ACOG) Committee on Obstetrics: Maternal and Fetal Medicine.

No woman should receive anticonvulsant medication unnecessarily. When possible, a woman who has been seizure free for many years should be withdrawn from her medication prior to pregnancy. When a woman who has epilepsy and requires medication asks about pregnancy, she should be advised that she has a 90% chance of having a normal child, but that the risk of congenital malformations and mental retardation is two to three times greater than average because of her disease or its treatment. . . .

There is no reason at present to advise a woman to switch from phenytoin or phenobarbital to other anticonvulsants about which even less is known. Discontinuation of medication in a woman whose epilepsy is controlled by medicine may cause seizures, and prolonged seizures could cause serious sequelae to her and the fetus.*

*From *Pediatrics* 63(2):331–333, Summary 333, February, 1979. Copyright American Academy of Pediatrics, 1979.

SPECIAL CONSIDERATIONS IN PREGNANCY

Phenobarbital rapidly crosses the placenta. It has been implicated as a possible teratogen causing cleft lip, congenital heart disease, and microcephaly. Thus far, the data are not conclusive.

Phenobarbital induces the production of fetal liver enzymes, including the glucuronyltransferase needed for bilirubin conjugation and excretion, and consequently has been recommended for both the prevention and treatment of neonatal hyperbilirubinemia. Enzyme induction is also associated with an increased rate of steroid metabolism and altered vitamin-D metabolism. Neonatal hypocalcemia has been reported. Coagulopathies resulting from a decrease in vitamin-K–dependent clotting factors have been seen in neonates following ingestion of phenobarbital by the mother. Withdrawal symptoms are commonly seen in neonates whose mothers have taken 90–120 mg of phenobarbital daily for at least 12 weeks prior to delivery.

Nursing mothers can usually take anticonvulsant doses of barbiturates without its affecting the infant. Drowsiness should be looked for in the nursing infant.

DOSAGE

In the treatment of epilepsy, the usual adult maintenance dose of phenobarbital is 60–300 mg (orally or parenterally) once daily. The therapeutic plasma concentration is 10–30 μg/ml. Dosage requirements increase during pregnancy. When phenobarbital is used as a mild sedative in preeclampsia, a dose of 30–60 mg is given every 6 hours, the higher dose being reserved for postpartum patients.

ADVERSE EFFECTS

Side effects include sedation, paradoxical irritability or hyperactivity in children, and confusion in the elderly. Nystagmus and ataxia are seen at excessive dosages. Megaloblastic anemia and osteomalacia have been associated with long-term phenobarbital therapy. Rare idiosyncratic reactions include scarlatiniform or morbilliform rashes, exfoliative dermatitis, agranulocytosis, and hepatitis.

MECHANISM OF ACTION

Phenobarbital increases the seizure threshold and limits the spread of seizure activity. These effects may be due to increased levels of gamma-aminobutyric acid, an inhibitory synaptic transmitter.

Barbiturates depress the activity of all excitable tissue, with the central nervous system being the most sensitive. There is little effect on skeletal, cardiac, or smooth muscle at therapeutic doses. By its combination with cytochrome P-450 and induction of hepatic microsomal enzymes, phenobarbital alters the metabolism of other drugs. The usual therapeutic range is 10–30 μg/ml.

ABSORPTION AND BIOTRANSFORMATION

Phenobarbital is well absorbed through the small intestine and from IM injection sites. Approximately 40%–60% of the drug is protein-bound. Ten to twenty-five percent is excreted unchanged in the urine; this process is enhanced by alkalinization and diuresis. The liver microsomal oxidizing system metabolizes the remaining drug, after which metabolites are excreted by the kidney. The half-life in adults is 2–6 days; it is longer in neonates and shorter in children.

RECOMMENDED READING

Anticonvulsants and pregnancy. Prepared by AAP Committee on Drugs in collaboration with the ACOG Committee on Obstetrics: Maternal and Fetal Medicine. January, 1979.

Eadie, M. J., and Tyrer, J. H. *Anticonvulsant Therapy.* Edinburgh: Churchill-Livingstone, 1974.

Friis, B., and Sardemann, H. Neonatal hypocalcemia after intrauterine exposure to anticonvulsant drugs. *Arch. Dis. Child.* 52:239–247, 1977.

Goodman, L. S., and Gilman, A. *The Pharmacological Basis of Therapeutics* (5th ed.). New York: Macmillan, 1975. Pp. 102–123, 209–210, 220.

Lander, C. M., Edwards, V. E., Eadie, M. J., and Tyrer, J. H. Plasma anticonvulsants concentration during pregnancy. *Neurology* 27:128–131, 1977.

Tuchmann-Duplessis, H. *Drug Effects on the Fetus.* Sydney, Australia: Adis Press, 1975.

Update: Drugs in breast milk. *Med. Lett. Drugs Ther.* 21:21, 1979.

Woodbury, D. M., Penry, J. K., and Schmidt, R. P. *Antiepileptic Drugs.* New York: Raven Press, 1972.

(PHR)

Phenols (over-the-counter)

INDICATIONS AND RECOMMENDATIONS

Phenols may be used safely during pregnancy in over-the-counter preparations containing dilute solutions. They should not be used in a strength greater than a 2% aqueous solution and also should not be used on broken skin.

These drugs are used as an antiseptic in mouthwashes as well as dermatological and anorectal preparations. Hexylresorcinol is the phenol most commonly used in mouthwashes. Thymol, while used in mouthwashes, is more frequently employed as a remedy for acne, hemorrhoids, and tinea pedis. Phenols have also been used alone or in combination with calamine lotion as an antipruritic agent.

SPECIAL CONSIDERATIONS IN PREGNANCY

No unusual maternal effects have been described during pregnancy, and no mutagenic or teratogenic effects have been reported. Convulsions, hepatic toxicity, and bone marrow depression are possible problems if toxic levels were to reach the fetus.

DOSAGE

Hexylresorcinol is used in a 1:1,000 concentration in mouthwashes. The various phenols are utilized in different concentrations, with all being absorbed to some degree.

ADVERSE EFFECTS

Significant skin penetration may occur when phenols are applied topically in solutions that are stronger than 2% aqueous or 4% in glycerin. This can result in tissue necrosis and systemic absorption. Erythema associated with some sloughing may occur. Cardiovascular effects include myocardial depression with secondary hypotension. Central nervous system action includes hypothermia. Ulceration of the stomach may occur if they are taken orally.

MECHANISM OF ACTION

Phenols are bacteriostatic as a 0.2% solution, bacteriocidal as a 1% solution, and fungicidal at 1.3% or greater. They combine with skin proteins to form a toxic substance. These drugs are more effective in an acid media, at higher temperatures, and in aqueous solution.

ABSORPTION AND BIOTRANSFORMATION

After being absorbed, about 80% is excreted by the kidney either unchanged or as a glucuronide. The remainder is oxidized to hydroquinone and pyrocatechol.

RECOMMENDED READING

Goodman, L. S., and Gilman, A. *The Pharmacological Basis of Therapeutics* (5th ed.). New York: Macmillan, 1975. Pp. 990–991.

Nelson, M. M., and Forfar, J. O.   Associations between drugs administered during pregnancy and congenital abnormalities of the fetus. *Br. Med. J.* 1:523–527, 1971.

Schenkel, B., and Vorherr, H.   Non-prescription drugs during pregnancy: Potential teratogenic and toxic effects upon embryo and fetus. *J. Reprod. Med.* 12:27–45, 1974.

(RAC)

Phenothiazines: Chlorpromazine (Thorazine®), Fluphenazine (Prolixin®), Perphenazine (Trilafon®), Prochlorperazine (Compazine®), Promethazine (Phenergan®), Thioridazine (Mellaril®), Trifluoperazine (Stelazine®)

INDICATIONS AND RECOMMENDATIONS

The use of phenothiazines during pregnancy should be limited to treatment of psychotic patients requiring continued medication. They are also used in the treatment of anxiety and restlessness, but safer alternatives are available. Drug therapy with phenothiazines should be discontinued 1 to 2 weeks prior to delivery to avoid symptoms in the neonate.

Prochlorperazine and promethazine are widely used as antiemetics. During pregnancy these drugs should be reserved for the treatment of severe nausea and vomiting. Bendectin®, a drug combination thoroughly evaluated in pregnancy, usually suffices for treatment of mild nausea and vomiting.

SPECIAL CONSIDERATIONS IN PREGNANCY

The phenothiazines theoretically pose a threat of maternal hypotension and consequent uteroplacental insufficiency. Antipsychotic medications are known to cross the placenta, and drug and metabolites have been identified in fetal plasma. In a review of over 6,000 pregnancies no increase in the incidence of malformations in a group of infants born to mothers who received chlorpromazine when compared to infants of controls was reported. Anecdotally, infants born to mothers who received phenothiazines during pregnancy have been reported to suffer from prolonged extrapyramidal effects, chromosomal anomalies, jaundice, mild sedation followed by motor excitement, agitation and hypertonicity, and depression.

Several studies have documented the presence of pheno-

163

thiazines in the breast milk of nursing mothers, but all state that no adverse effects have been noted in mother or infant. The quantities excreted in breast milk are very small, only 0.29 μg/ml having been measured 2 hours after a single 1,200 mg dose of chlorpromazine.

DOSAGE

Phenothiazine dosage should be individualized according to the severity of the condition, the patient's age, and the clinical response. It should be administered in divided doses during the first few weeks of therapy, but thereafter may be administered in a once-daily or twice-daily regimen. Fluphenazine is also available in injectable forms that may be administered every 2 weeks. Table 11 details the recommended doses of some of the phenothiazines.

When used as an antiemetic, prochlorperazine may be given as an oral tablet (5 or 10 mg) every 4–6 hours, or as a rectal suppository, 25 mg every 12 hours. The intramuscular dose is 5–10 mg every 6 hours. Promethazine is given orally or rectally, 25–50 mg daily, or intramuscularly, 12.5–25 mg every 4–6 hours.

ADVERSE EFFECTS

The most frequent side effects of the phenothiazines are drowsiness; postural hypotension; and anticholinergic effects, including dry mouth, constipation, mydriasis and cycloplegia, urinary retention, and tachycardia. These appear early in the treatment course, and patients usually develop a tolerance to them. Because phenothiazines depress the mechanism for heat regulation they may cause hyperthermia or hypothermia, depending on ambient

Table 11. Dosage Range of Phenothiazines[a] (for Psychosis)

Drug	Usual Daily Dosage Range, Oral or IM (mg)	Maximum Daily Dose (mg)
Chlorpromazine	50–800	2,000
Fluphenazine	2.5–20	40
Perphenazine	8–24	64
Thioridazine[b]	50–600	800
Trifluoperazine	2–15	64

[a]Prochlorperazine and promethazine are discussed in more detail in the text.
[b]Only given orally.

temperature. Parkinsonism, dystonia, galactorrhea, photosensitivity, menstrual changes, and blood dyscrasias have also been noted occasionally with their use.

MECHANISM OF ACTION

The mechanisms of action of the phenothiazines are only partly known. Their effects may be due to blockage of dopamine receptors and dopamine release in the caudate nucleus, and to inhibition of the dopamine activation of adenyl cyclase. In the brain stem, the inflow of stimuli to the reticular formation is selectively decreased. Most phenothiazine derivatives exert a depressant action on the chemoreceptor trigger zone, thereby suppressing emesis due to conditions in which this center is stimulated.

Antipsychotic agents have peripheral anticholinergic activity and alpha-adrenergic blocking activity. They can inhibit the release of growth hormone and may antagonize secretion of prolactin-release inhibiting hormone, producing galactorrhea. They can lower the convulsive threshold and may interfere with temperature regulation.

ABSORPTION AND BIOTRANSFORMATION

The phenothiazines are generally rapidly absorbed from the gastrointestinal tract and from parenteral injection sites. They are highly soluble and strongly bound to plasma proteins. Inactivation occurs largely through oxidation by hepatic microsomal enzymes.

RECOMMENDED READING

AMA Drug Evaluations (3rd ed.).   Littleton, Mass.: Publishing Sciences Group, 1977. Pp. 420–451, 1090–1105.

American Hospital Formulary Service. *Monograph on Phenothiazines.* Washington, D.C.: American Society of Hospital Pharmacists, 1977.

Ayd, F. J., Jr.   Excretion of psychotropic drugs in human breast milk. *Int. Drug Ther. Newslett.* 8:33–40, 1973.

Baldessarini, R. J.   *Chemotherapy in Psychiatry.* Cambridge: Harvard University Press, 1977. Pp. 12–56.

Drugs for psychiatric disorders.   *Med. Lett. Drugs Ther.* 18:89–96, 1976.

Goodman, L. S., and Gilman, A.   *The Pharmacological Basis of Therapeutics* (5th ed.). New York: Macmillan, 1975. Pp. 152–174.

(CRS)

Phenoxybenzamine (Dibenzyline®)

INDICATIONS AND RECOMMENDATIONS

The use of phenoxybenzamine during pregnancy should be limited to the treatment of hypertension due to pheochromocytoma. Acute hypertensive *crises* associated with pheochromocytoma, however, should be controlled with intravenous phentolamine. Phenoxybenzamine then becomes the drug of choice for oral maintenance therapy. Control of blood pressure during cesarean section or during surgery to remove the tumor should also be maintained with intravenous phentolamine.

SPECIAL CONSIDERATIONS IN PREGNANCY

Untreated pheochromocytoma during pregnancy has been associated with maternal and fetal mortality rates of up to 48% and 47%, respectively. It is presumed that most of these deaths were due to maternal cardiovascular problems that led to fetal anoxia. Phenoxybenzamine has been used successfully in the last trimester of pregnancy for the treatment of hypertension secondary to pheochromocytoma.

One case of premature rupture of the membranes following 3 days of phenoxybenzamine therapy in the twenty-sixth week of pregnancy has been reported. The subsequent hypertensive crisis was controlled by phentolamine. A 640-gm infant was born 21 hours later and died shortly thereafter. One instance of maternal and fetal tachycardia following parenteral administration of phenoxybenzamine has been reported. The child was normal at follow-up 8 years later.

DOSAGE

Only the oral form of phenoxybenzamine is currently available for use in the United States. The usual oral dose is 10 mg once a day initially; it can then be raised by 10 mg increments every 4 days until the desired response is obtained. At least 2 weeks are usually required to reach the optimal dosage.

ADVERSE EFFECTS

The most frequently noticed side effects are due to alpha-adrenergic blockade and vary with the degree of blockade. These include postural hypotension, reflex tachycardia, miosis, and nasal congestion. Sedation, nausea, and vomiting are also seen. Patients with hypovolemia may suffer from a sharp fall in blood pressure when this drug is administered.

MECHANISM OF ACTION

Phenoxybenzamine produces alpha-adrenergic blockade by establishing stable bonds at receptor sites, thus reducing the total population of available alpha receptors and decreasing responses mediated by their excessive stimulation. Beta-adrenergic stimulation is consequently unopposed. Vasodilation in various vascular beds depends in part upon the degrees of alpha-adrenergic and beta-adrenergic control.

Normal subjects who are standing and receive phenoxybenzamine slowly by the intravenous route show little change in blood pressure, although diastolic values tend to fall; in normal recumbent subjects, however, a precipitous fall in blood pressure occurs. Cerebral and coronary vascular resistance is not altered greatly. Hypertension due to excessive catecholamine production in patients with pheochromocytoma can be controlled by the oral administration of phenoxybenzamine.

ABSORPTION AND BIOTRANSFORMATION

Twenty to thirty percent of an oral dose of phenoxybenzamine is absorbed from the gastrointestinal tract. The drug is primarily excreted in the urine, with 50% being eliminated in the first 12 hours and 80% in 24 hours.

RECOMMENDED READING

Brenner, W. E., Yen, S. S., Dingfelder, J. R., and Anton, A. H. Pheochromocytoma: Serial studies during pregnancy. *Am. J. Obstet. Gynecol.* 113:779–788, 1972.

Goodman, L. S., and Gilman, A. *The Pharmacological Basis of Therapeutics* (5th ed.). New York: Macmillan, 1975. Pp. 533–540.

Griffith, M. I., Felts, J. H., James, F. M., Meyers, R. T., Shealy, G. M., and Woodruff, L. F. Successful control of pheochromocytoma in pregnancy. *J.A.M.A.* 229:437–439, 1974.

Leak, D., Carroll, J. J., Robinson, D. C., and Ashworth, E. J. Management of pheochromocytoma during pregnancy. *Can. Med. Assoc. J.* 116:371–375, 1977.

Maughan, G. B., Shabanah, E. H., and Toth, A. Experiments with pharmacologic sympatholysis in the gravid. *Am. J. Obstet. Gynecol.* 97:764–776, 1967.

(BDH)

Phentolamine (Regitine®)

INDICATIONS AND RECOMMENDATIONS

The use of phentolamine during pregnancy should be limited to the treatment of acute hypertensive episodes in patients with pheochromocytoma and for the immediate preoperative and intraoperative management of such a patient undergoing cesarean section for delivery of the infant and removal of the tumor. Both mother and fetus should be monitored carefully during the procedure. It is not recommended as a diagnostic agent in, or for chronic management of, pheochromocytoma in pregnancy.

SPECIAL CONSIDERATIONS IN PREGNANCY

It is not recommended that phentolamine be used as a diagnostic agent for pheochromocytoma in the pregnant patient, since a severe drop in maternal blood pressure will cause decreased uterine blood flow and corresponding fetal anoxia. Safer diagnostic tests such as bioassays and chemical assays for catecholamines are available.

Phenoxybenzamine is the agent of choice for preoperative management of pheochromocytoma. Phentolamine, however, is given intravenously for the control of hypertension during delivery and tumor removal. One case of a baby born with "jitters" following treatment of the mother with phentolamine and guanethidine has been reported.

DOSAGE

For use in preoperative reduction of elevated blood pressure, 5 mg intravenously or intramuscularly is given 1–2 hours before surgery and repeated if necessary. During surgery, 5 mg may be administered intravenously to prevent or control paroxysms of hypertension, tachycardia, or other effects of epinephrine intoxication. The 5-mg dose is also used for treatment of acute hypertensive crises and may be repeated as necessary. Blood pressure should be monitored frequently for 10 minutes after injection. Norepinephrine should be on hand to reverse any hypotension.

ADVERSE EFFECTS

The primary side effects of phentolamine are caused by gastrointestinal and cardiac stimulation. Gastrointestinal symptoms include pain, nausea, vomiting, diarrhea, and exacerbation of peptic ulcer. Cardiac stimulation may lead to tachycardia, angina, and cardiac arrhythmias, especially after parenteral administration. Death due to hypoglycemia has been observed with chronic overdosage.

MECHANISM OF ACTION

Phentolamine is a moderately effective alpha-adrenergic blocker; vasodilation produced at doses usually used in adults, however, results primarily from its direct effect on vascular smooth muscle. Only high doses produce characteristic alpha-adrenergic blockade. The drug increases circulatory catecholamines in normal patients.

Clinical manifestations of pheochromocytoma result from the secretion of catecholamines. Vasodilation produced by phentolamine causes a fall in blood pressure, especially in patients with pheochromocytoma. The hypotension may be potentially severe in such patients.

ABSORPTION AND BIOTRANSFORMATION

Phentolamine is absorbed after oral administration, but the drug is less than 20% as active when given orally than when given by parenteral administration. Approximately 10% of an intravenous dose is recovered unchanged in the urine. The fate of the remaining drug is unknown.

RECOMMENDED READING

Brenner, W. E., Yen, S. S., Dingfelder, J. R., and Anton, A. H. Pheochromocytoma: Serial studies during pregnancy. *Am. J. Obstet. Gynecol.* 113:779–788, 1972.

Griffith, M. I., Felts, J. H., James, F. M., Meyers, R. T., Shealy, G. M., and Woodruff, L. F. Successful control of pheochromocytoma in pregnancy. *J.A.M.A.* 229:437–439, 1974.

Leak, D., Carroll, J. J., and Robinson, D. C. Management of pheochromocytoma during pregnancy. *Can. Med. Assoc. J.* 116:371–375, 1977.

Maughan, G. B., Shabanah, E. H., and Toth, A. Experiments with pharmacologic sympatholysis in the gravid. *Am. J. Obstet. Gynecol.* 97:764–776, 1967.

(BDH)

Phenylbutazone (Butazolidin®)

INDICATIONS AND RECOMMENDATIONS

The use of phenylbutazone should be limited to a 4-day course of treatment for an attack of acute gouty arthritis. Gout is uncommon in women and rarely seen before menopause. If treatment of an acute attack becomes necessary during pregnancy, a *short* course of phenylbutazone is preferable to the use of colchicine or allopurinol. Monitoring blood counts, serum electrolytes, and fluid balance is mandatory. This drug is a potent anti-inflammatory agent, a poor analgesic, and a weak antipyretic agent. It is contraindicated for the treatment of rheumatoid arthritis and allied disorders during pregnancy because aspirin or corticosteroids are preferable therapeutic agents.

SPECIAL CONSIDERATIONS IN PREGNANCY

Phenylbutazone causes marked sodium and water retention accompanied by decreased urinary output and increased plasma volume up to 50%. Since plasma volume in pregnancy is already expanded, cardiac decompensation could result from the administration of this drug.

The risk of teratogenesis in humans is unknown. The package insert states that animal studies, though inconclusive thus far, exhibit evidence of embryotoxicity.

DOSAGE

The recommended dose to be used for an attack of gouty arthritis is 200 mg by mouth qid for the first day followed by 100 mg by mouth tid for 3 additional days.

ADVERSE EFFECTS

Some type of side effect is noted in 10% to 45% of patients taking this drug. Side effects include nausea, vomiting, epigastric discomfort, skin rashes, diarrhea, vertigo, insomnia, euphoria, nervousness, and edema formation. More serious adverse sequelae include peptic ulceration with hemorrhage or perforation, serum-sickness-like hypersensitivity reactions, hepatitis, nephritis, and the particularly dangerous possibility of bone marrow suppression with aplastic anemia, leukopenia, agranulocytosis, and/or thrombocytopenia. A number of patients have died from the aplastic anemia and agranulocytosis. There is also a well-documented increased risk of bleeding when phenylbutazone is given to a patient receiving warfarin anticoagulant therapy.

MECHANISM OF ACTION

The mechanism of action of the anti-inflammatory effects of phenylbutazone is not known. Like the salicylates, this drug inhibits the biosynthesis of prostaglandins, uncouples oxidative phosphorylation, and inhibits the adenosine triphosphate (ATP)-dependent biosynthesis of mucopolysaccharide sulfates in cartilage. The uricosuric effect results from diminished tubular reabsorption of uric acid. Sodium and chloride retention also results from a direct effect on the renal tubules. The excretion of potassium is not changed. Phenylbutazone reduces iodine uptake by the thyroid gland by a direct action that inhibits the synthesis of organic iodine compounds.

Other anti-inflammatory drugs, oral anticoagulants, oral hypoglycemic agents, sulfonamides, and some other drugs may be displaced from binding proteins by phenylbutazone. This can result in an increased pharmacological or toxic effect of the displaced drug.

ABSORPTION AND BIOTRANSFORMATION

Phenylbutazone is rapidly absorbed from the gastrointestinal tract, and peak levels are reached in 2 hours. The drug is 98% bound to plasma proteins, and the serum half-life is 50–100 hours.

Phenylbutazone is almost entirely metabolized in the liver. Oxyphenbutazone, one of the two metabolites, has pharmacological and toxic properties similar to the parent compound. Both phenylbutazone and oxyphenbutazone are slowly excreted in the urine, since binding to plasma proteins limits their glomerular filtration. Because of their slow metabolism and excretion, these compounds may accumulate in considerable quantities during long-term administration.

RECOMMENDED READING

Burrow, G. N., and Ferris, T. F. (Eds.). *Medical Complications During Pregnancy*. New York: W.B. Saunders, 1975. P. 805.

Goldfinger, S. E. Treatment of gout. *N. Engl. J. Med.* 285:1303–1306, 1971.

Goodman, L. S., and Gilman, A. *The Pharmacological Basis of Therapeutics* (5th ed.). New York: Macmillan, 1975. Pp. 350–352.

(RLB)

Phenytoin (Dilantin®)

INDICATIONS AND RECOMMENDATIONS

The use of phenytoin during pregnancy should be limited to the treatment of those women requiring anticonvulsant therapy. The following recommendations have been made in a bulletin published in 1979 by the American Academy of Pediatrics Committee on Drugs in collaboration with the American College of Obstetrics and Gynecology (ACOG) Committee on Obstetrics: Maternal and Fetal Medicine.

No woman should receive anticonvulsant medication unnecessarily. When possible, a woman who has been seizure free for many years should be withdrawn from her medication prior to pregnancy. When a woman who has epilepsy and requires medication asks about pregnancy, she should be advised that she has a 90% chance of having a normal child, but that the risk of congenital malformations and mental retardation is two to three times greater than average because of her disease or its treatment. Women who seek advice later than the first trimester of pregnancy should be reassured with the foregoing figures rather than routinely urged to consider abortion. For these women, drug therapy should be continued throughout pregnancy because major anatomical malformations most likely would have taken place already, and the malformations associated with the hydantoin syndrome rarely have significant effect on the well-being of the child.

There is no reason at present to advise a woman to switch from phenytoin or phenobarbital to other anticonvulsants about which even less is known. Discontinuation of medication in a woman whose epilepsy is controlled by medicine may cause seizures, and prolonged seizures could cause serious sequelae to her and the fetus.*

Phenytoin is most commonly used as an anticonvulsant in the treatment of grand mal, status epilepticus, focal motor, sensory, and psychomotor seizures. It is also, more rarely, used as an intravenous antiarrhythmic agent in the treatment of ventricular arrhythmias, but alternative agents for this are preferred during pregnancy.

At delivery, measurement of cord blood calcium and prothrombin time followed by vitamin-K administration are indicated. Neonatal glucose levels should be checked shortly after birth. Breastfeeding is not contraindicated.

*From *Pediatrics* 63(2):331–333, summary 333, February, 1979. Copyright American Academy of Pediatrics, 1979.

SPECIAL CONSIDERATIONS IN PREGNANCY

Dosage requirements for phenytoin have been reported by one author to increase during pregnancy and fall in the puerperium, although this remains controversial. Phenytoin readily crosses the placenta, and identical maternal and fetal plasma levels have been reported at delivery. Elimination of the drug by the full-term neonate has been shown to be similar to that of adults.

Phenytoin teratogenicity and mutagenicity have been demonstrated in rats and mice but not in monkeys. There is an increased risk of congenital heart disease and cleft palate among the offspring of women with epilepsy, most of whom are on anticonvulsants. Part of this increase may be caused by phenytoin. The risk of all abnormalities in these infants appears to be about 4% to 5%, which is approximately double the rate of malformations in the general population. Recent reports have described a combination of defects, the fetal hydantoin syndrome, felt to be secondary to phenytoin. The syndrome consists of craniofacial anomalies, intrauterine growth retardation, mental retardation, and nail and digital hypoplasia. It is associated with fetal exposure to phenytoin, although it has not been proved to be caused by the drug. The risk of this syndrome is of unknown magnitude, but it is probably less than 10%. As with phenobarbital, phenytoin has been associated with a vitamin-K–deficient coagulopathy in the neonate.

DOSAGE

The usual adult maintenance dose of phenytoin in anticonvulsant therapy is about 300 mg daily or 3.5 mg/kg/day. This dosage should produce serum levels in the therapeutic range of 10–20 μg/ml. As the half-life of phenytoin is relatively long, steady state serum levels are reached in 6–10 days when no loading dose is given. These can be reached more quickly if a load of 1,000 mg in divided doses over 1–2 days is given prior to institution of maintenance therapy. Dosage alterations should await achievement of a plateau level and should be attempted in small stepwise increments since phenytoin exhibits dose-dependent kinetics; dosage increases may lead to larger than expected increases in serum levels.

Intravenous therapy is sometimes indicated when a patient is not able to take oral medications and in the treatment of status epilepticus and ventricular arrhythmias. Phenytoin should not be given intramuscularly since the drug is erratically absorbed from the site of administration. The drug should be administered at a rate not greater than 50 mg/min and should not be diluted since it may crystallize out of solution.

Changes in the serum phenytoin level secondary to drug interactions may adversely affect the therapeutic response. Carbamazepine may decrease steady state phenytoin levels while isoniazid and chloramphenicol may increase such levels. When phenobarbital is given concurrently, it may either increase or decrease phenytoin plasma concentrations by either increasing or competitively inhibiting its metabolism.

ADVERSE EFFECTS

Idiosyncratic reactions to phenytoin include skin rashes, exfoliative dermatitis, lymphadenopathy, fever, systemic lupus erythematosus, pancytopenia or a decrease in isolated blood cell types, and a lymphoma-like syndrome. Long-term use of phenytoin at therapeutic doses may result in gingival hyperplasia, hirsutism, decreased insulin secretion with resultant hyperglycemia and glucosuria, osteomalacia with hypocalcemia, and megaloblastic anemia due to altered folate metabolism.

When phenytoin serum levels exceed the recommended 10–20 μg/ml, cerebellar-vestibular effects may be noticed. These include nystagmus, ataxia, vertigo, and diplopia. Cardiovascular collapse or central nervous system depression, or both, may be seen when phenytoin is administered intravenously at a rate greater than 50 mg/min.

MECHANISM OF ACTION

Phenytoin blocks the spread of electrical activity from the seizure focus by stabilizing the neuronal membrane and preventing post-tetanic potentiation. It is effective in the treatment of grand mal, focal motor, and psychomotor seizures, but it can exacerbate petit mal seizures.

Its cardiac antiarrhythmic effect is related to a reduction in both action potential duration (APD) and effective refractory period (ERP) but an increase in the ERP to ADP ratio. Ventricular automaticity is decreased and atrioventricular conduction increased. Myocardial contractile force and blood pressure are lowered. The degree of hypotension and cardiac depression seems to be related to dose and speed of injection and may be due to propylene glycol, a solubilizing agent in the intravenous solution.

ABSORPTION AND BIOTRANSFORMATION

Phenytoin is absorbed through the duodenum and readily bound to albumin and alpha-globulins. The plasma protein binding is not significantly altered in pregnancy. Phenytoin is hydroxylated to an inactive metabolite by the liver; the metabolite is excreted via the kidneys. The rate of metabolism is variable, with a half-life usually ranging from 17–56 hours.

RECOMMENDED READING

Anticonvulsants and pregnancy. Prepared by the AAP Committee on Drugs in collaboration with the ACOG Committee on Obstetrics: Maternal and Fetal Medicine. January, 1979.

Eadie, M. J., and Tyrer, J. H. *Anticonvulsant Therapy*. Edinburgh: Churchill-Livingstone, 1974.

Goodman, L. S., and Gilman, A. *The Pharmacological Basis of Therapeutics* (5th ed.). New York: Macmillan, 1975. Pp. 204–208, 697–698.

Lander, C. M., Edwards, V. E., Eadie, M. J., and Tyrer, J. H. Plasma anticonvulsant concentrations during pregnancy. *Neurology* (Minneap.) 27:128–131, 1977.

Mirkin, B. L. Diphenylhydantoin: Placental transport, fetal localization, neonatal metabolism, and possible teratogenic effects. *J. Pediatr.* 78:329–337, 1971.

Tuchmann-Duplessis, H. *Drug Effects on the Fetus*. Sydney, Australia: Adis Press, 1975.

Woodbury, D. M., Penry, J. K., and Schmidt, R. P. *Antiepileptic Drugs*. New York: Raven Press, 1972.

(PHR)

Potassium Chloride, Oral (K-Lor®, K-Lyte/Cl®, Kaochlor®, Slow-K®)

INDICATIONS AND RECOMMENDATIONS

Oral potassium chloride is safe to use during pregnancy. It is indicated for treatment or prophylaxis of potassium deficiency. Serum potassium levels should be followed when this compound is administered. It will almost certainly be necessary to prescribe potassium chloride when a pregnant woman is taking thiazide diuretics for control of hypertension.

SPECIAL CONSIDERATIONS IN PREGNANCY

Fetal potassium levels are dependent upon maternal potassium levels. Fetal bradycardia due to heart block has been reported in association with hypokalemia in the mother.

DOSAGE

The usual daily dose is 80 mEq over 24 hours. Oral potassium should be taken with a full glass of water or orange juice. Measurement of serial serum potassium levels should be used to monitor efficacy of therapy. The chloride salt of potassium should be given since failure to replace chloride will enhance the potassium loss in metabolic alkalosis.

Potassium chloride is available in a variety of dosage forms, including liquids in 10% (20 mEq/15 ml) and 20% (40 mEq/15 ml) strengths; powders providing 15 mEq, 20 mEq, and 25 mEq per dose; and wax matrix tablets in 500 or 600 mg strengths. Although enteric-coated tablets are available, their use is not recommended as they are associated with an increased incidence of intestinal ulceration.

ADVERSE EFFECTS

Side effects of excessive oral potassium supplementation include vomiting, diarrhea, nausea, and abdominal discomfort. Toxicity is most likely to occur in conditions such as oliguria, azotemia, acute dehydration, and untreated Addison's disease. Manifestations of toxicity include paresthesias of the extremities, flaccid paralysis, listlessness, mental confusion, weakness, and decrease in blood pressure. Electrocardiographic changes include loss of the P wave, widening of the QRS complex, ST segment changes, and tall peaked T waves.

MECHANISM OF ACTION

The mechanism of action of potassium on skeletal, cardiac, and smooth muscle, and its renal and metabolic effects, are beyond the scope of this book. The reader is referred to a current textbook of physiology.

Causes of potassium deficiency include diarrhea, vomiting, decreased intake, increased renal excretion (as in diuresis, acidosis, or adrenocortical hyperactivity), increased cellular uptake (as in treatment of diabetic ketoacidosis), persistent alkalosis, and familial periodic paralysis.

RECOMMENDED READING

Goodman, L. S., and Gilman, A. *The Pharmacological Basis of Therapeutics* (5th ed.). New York: Macmillan, 1975. P. 974.

(GRD)

Potassium Iodide

INDICATIONS AND RECOMMENDATIONS

The use of potassium iodide is contraindicated in pregnancy. It has been used as an expectorant in the form of a solution or pill. It is contraindicated in pregnancy because of the potential for formation of fetal goiter secondary to fetal thyroid trapping of the iodide.

RECOMMENDED READING

Carswell, F., Kerr, M. M., and Hutchison, J. H. Congenital goitre and hypothyroidism produced by maternal ingestion of iodides. *Lancet* 1:1241–1243, 1970.

(GRD)

Primidone (Mysoline®)

INDICATIONS AND RECOMMENDATIONS

The use of primidone during pregnancy should be limited to the treatment of those women requiring chronic anticonvulsant therapy. It is used alone or in combination with other anticonvulsants for the treatment of generalized tonic-clonic, cortical focal, or temporal lobe epilepsy. Primidone may be given to breastfeeding mothers, but the nursing infant should be observed for drowsiness.

The following recommendations have been made in a bulletin published in 1979 by the American Academy of Pediatrics Committee on Drugs in collaboration with the American College of Obstetrics and Gynecology (ACOG) Committee on Obstetrics: Maternal and Fetal Medicine.

No woman should receive anticonvulsant medication unnecessarily. When possible, a woman who has been seizure free for many years should be withdrawn from her medication prior to pregnancy. When a woman who has epilepsy and requires medication asks about pregnancy, she should be advised that she has a 90% chance of having a normal child, but that the risk of congenital malformations and mental retardation is two to three times greater than average because of her disease or its treatment.*

*From *Pediatrics* 63(2):331–333, summary 333, February, 1979. Copyright American Academy of Pediatrics, 1979.

SPECIAL CONSIDERATIONS IN PREGNANCY

Primidone crosses the placenta, and it has been cited as a possible cause of birth anomalies. Reported incidents in past years, however, have been inconclusive in light of the practice of multi-drug therapy for epilepsy.

Offspring of pregnant mice receiving 25–150 mg/kg/day of primidone exhibited a high incidence of palatal defects, including full-length and submucosal clefts. No strong dose-dependence was found in association with the abnormalities. The mice demonstrated the same metabolites as those found in man. Administered doses were not much larger, on a mg/kg basis, than those used in humans.

When primidone was the sole anticonvulsant agent used in 3 pregnant women, it was found that 2 of the 3 infants born to these women had a cleft palate. The third infant had no congenital anomalies. Another report on a mother who received only primidone during her pregnancy described the infant as having fragile primary teeth, hypoplasia of distal phalanges and nails, and stunted length (below the 16th percentile).

In addition to the gross defects found at birth, reports exist that describe a withdrawal-like syndrome in some otherwise normal infants born to mothers receiving daily doses of primidone. In two reports, the infants were tremulous and irritable for 3 days, cord blood contained 8 μg/ml of primidone, and the drug could be detected in the infants' urine for 10–11 days. Hypoprothrombinemia has been reported in infants of mothers on a combination of primidone and phenobarbital. It is not conclusive that primidone alone can decrease prothrombin levels, but as it is metabolized to phenobarbital, this is possible. The condition usually responds to vitamin-K therapy.

The manufacturers recommend that mothers taking primidone discontinue nursing if the infant appears unusually drowsy.

DOSAGE

The usual adult oral dose is 500–1,500 mg per day given in divided doses. The dosage is adjusted primarily on the basis of the resulting phenobarbital concentration. Primidone concentration can also be monitored but is less reliable. The plasma phenobarbital concentration averages 2 μg/ml per mg/kg of primidone while plasma primidone concentration averages 1 μg/ml per mg/kg of primidone. Phenobarbital serum concentrations in the usual therapeutic range of 10–20 μg/ml are sought.

ADVERSE EFFECTS

The side effects of primidone are similar to those of phenobarbital and include sedation, vertigo, dizziness, ataxia, diplopia, nystagmus, megaloblastic anemia, and possibly osteomalacia. Idiosyncratic reactions include skin rashes, leukopenia, thrombocytopenia, lymphadenopathy, and a systemic lupus erthematosus-like syndrome.

MECHANISM OF ACTION

The mechanism of action of primidone is complex due to the presence of two active metabolites, phenobarbital and phenylethylmalonamide (PEMA) in addition to the drug itself. In rat studies PEMA has been shown to raise the thresholds for myoclonic jerks and clonic-tonic seizures induced by hexafluorodiethylether. In studies of electroconvulsion, in both man and animals primidone appears more selective than phenobarbital alone in controlling certain phases of seizure activity. (See *Phenobarbital* for its actions.)

Primidone is useful in the control of generalized tonic-clonic, cortical focal, and temporal lobe epilepsy. Patients whose conditions are refractory to other anticonvulsants may respond to primidone alone; however, it is commonly used in conjunction with phenytoin with increased efficacy. As primidone is metabolized to phenobarbital, the use of these two drugs concurrently is irrational.

ABSORPTION AND BIOTRANSFORMATION

The drug is rapidly absorbed through the gastrointestinal tract and is metabolized in the liver to the active compounds, PEMA and phenobarbital. Primidone's plasma half-life is less than 10 hours. PEMA appears rapidly and has a half-life of 2–6 days. Unaltered primidone and presumably PEMA are excreted by the kidneys.

RECOMMENDED READING

Anticonvulsants and pregnancy. Prepared by the AAP Committee on Drugs in collaboration with the ACOG Committee on Obstetrics: Maternal and Fetal Medicine. January, 1979.

Eadie, M. J., and Tyrer, J. H. *Anticonvulsant Therapy.* Edinburgh: Churchill-Livingstone, 1974.

Friis, B., and Sardemann, H. Neonatal hypocalcemia after intrauterine exposure to anticonvulsant drugs. *Arch. Dis. Child.* 52:239–241, 1977.

Goodman, L. S., and Gilman, A. *The Pharmacological Basis of Therapeutics* (5th ed.). New York: Macmillan, 1975. Pp. 210–211.

Martinez, G., and Snyder, R. D. Transplacental passage of primidone. *Neurology* 23:381–383, 1973.

Mygind, K. I., Dam, M., and Christiansen, J.   Phenytoin and phenobarbitone plasma clearance during pregnancy. *Acta Neurol. Scand.* 54:160–166, 1976.

Update: Drugs in breast milk.   *Med. Lett. Drugs Ther.* 21:21–24, 1979.

Woodbury, D. M., Penry, J. K., and Schmidt, R. P.   *Antiepileptic Drugs.* New York: Raven Press, 1972.

(ADD)

Probenecid (Benemid®)

INDICATIONS AND RECOMMENDATIONS

The use of probenecid during pregnancy should be limited to the treatment of gout or potentially symptomatic hyperuricemia. Since it has no analgesic or anti-inflammatory activity, it is of no value in the treatment of acute attacks of gout and phenylbutazone may be used in these instances. Probenecid is commonly given before the administration of penicillin or ampicillin, especially in the treatment of gonorrheal infections, to increase blood levels of the antibiotics by inhibiting their renal excretion. It would seem judicious to avoid using two drugs in pregnancy if one would suffice.

SPECIAL CONSIDERATIONS IN PREGNANCY

Probenecid is known to cross the placental barrier. With the exception of the death of 1 neonate not definitely related to probenecid therapy, the drug has been used in pregnancy without adverse effect to mother or child.

DOSAGE

Therapy should not be started until 2 to 3 weeks after an acute attack. The usual dose is 250 mg bid for 1 week followed by 500 mg bid. Daily dosage may be increased every 4 weeks by increments of 500 mg to a maximum of 2–3 gm.

ADVERSE EFFECTS

Frequently reported side effects include headache, anorexia, nausea, and vomiting. Dizziness, flushing, sore gums, urinary frequency, and anemia have also been reported. Probenecid therapy may exacerbate and prolong inflammation during the acute phase of gout. The frequency of attacks may also be increased during the first 6–12 weeks of therapy.

MECHANISM OF ACTION

Renal transport of organic acids is influenced by probenecid therapy. It is a competitive inhibitor to active reabsorption of uric acid at the proximal convoluted tubule. Urinary excretion of uric acid is therefore increased and serum urate levels are reduced. Subtherapeutic doses may inhibit renal secretion of uric acid.

At the proximal and distal tubules, probenecid competitively inhibits secretion of many weak organic acids such as the penicillins. Plasma levels of acidic drugs primarily eliminated by tubular secretion can be substantially increased.

By decreasing serum urate levels, probenecid prevents or reduces chronic joint changes and tophi formation. It eventually reduces the frequency of attacks and may improve renal function in gouty patients. Serum urate levels usually reach a minimum within a few days after therapy is begun.

ABSORPTION AND BIOTRANSFORMATION

Probenecid is rapidly and completely absorbed from the gastrointestinal tract. Following oral administration of 2 gm, plasma half-life ranges from 4–17 hours and decreases as the dose decreases. Approximately 75% of the drug is bound to plasma proteins. Probenecid is metabolized in the liver.

RECOMMENDED READING

American Hospital Formulary Service. *Monographs for Allopurinol* (1977), *Colchicine* (1973), and *Probenecid* (1977). Washington, D.C.: American Society of Hospital Pharmacists, 1973, 1977.

Burrow, G. N., and Ferris, T. F. *Medical Complications During Pregnancy*. New York: Saunders, 1975.

Goodman, L. S., and Gilman, A. *The Pharmacological Basis of Therapeutics* (5th ed.). New York: Macmillan, 1975. Pp. 862–863.

Lee, F. I., and Loeffler, F. E. Gout and pregnancy. *J. Obstet. Gynaecol. Br. Commonw.* 69:299–304, 1962.

(CRV)

Procainamide (Pronestyl®)

INDICATIONS AND RECOMMENDATIONS

The use of procainamide in pregnancy should be limited to the treatment of those patients with cardiac arrhythmias that are unresponsive to safer antiarrhythmic agents. Quinidine, with its similar electrophysiological effects, is preferred during pregnancy because it has been more extensively studied.

SPECIAL CONSIDERATIONS IN PREGNANCY

Little is known about the use of procainamide during pregnancy.

DOSAGE

The usual oral maintenance dose is 6 mg/kg every 3 hours. When given intravenously the dose is 200–500 mg administered at a rate not exceeding 25–50 mg/min, followed by a maintenance infusion of 2 mg/kg/hour. The therapeutic range is 4–8 μg/ml.

ADVERSE EFFECTS

The use of procainamide is often accompanied by prolongation of the QRS interval on electrocardiogram and by hypotension. Ventricular tachycardia and heart block may be seen with toxic doses (greater than 12 μg/ml). Besides these electrophysiological side effects, chronic administration of procainamide is associated with a systemic lupus erythematosus-like syndrome. Most patients on long-term therapy develop a positive antinuclear antibody titer, although few show a complete lupus syndrome.

MECHANISM OF ACTION

Procainamide decreases cardiac membrane responsiveness. Automaticity and speed of impulse conduction are therefore decreased, and the refractory period is increased.

ABSORPTION AND BIOTRANSFORMATION

Procainamide is rapidly and almost completely absorbed from the gastrointestinal tract. Maximal plasma concentration after oral administration occurs at about 60 minutes, and at 15–60 minutes after intramuscular administration. Procainamide has a half-life of 2½–5 hours in patients with normal renal function. It is acetylated in the liver to N-acetylprocainamide (NAPA), a compound that also possesses antiarrhythmic activity. The rate of acetylation of procainamide is genetically determined and varies among individuals. The half-life of NAPA is 7 hours in patients with normal renal function. The total amount of unchanged procainamide excreted in the urine varies from 40%–70% and depends upon acetylator phenotype.

RECOMMENDED READING

Avery, G. S. *Drug Treatment: Principles and Practice of Clinical Pharmacology and Therapeutics.* Sydney, Australia: Adis Press, 1976.
Goodman, L. S., and Gilman, A. *The Pharmacological Basis of Therapeutics* (5th ed.). New York: Macmillan, 1975. Pp. 694–696.

(MJM)

Progestins

Natural Progesterone and Its Esters (Delalutin®, Provera®)

INDICATIONS AND RECOMMENDATIONS

The use of progesterone and its esters, 17-hydroxyprogesterone, medroxyprogesterone acetate (Provera®) and 17-hydroxyprogesterone caproate (Delalutin®) during pregnancy is controversial and if used at all should be restricted to very specific situations.

Natural progesterone can probably be given safely during pregnancy for the treatment of an inadequate luteal phase, and along with its esters for the prevention of premature delivery. The efficacy of these agents is still open to question, however. There is no convincing evidence that progesterone in any form is useful in the management of threatened abortion or habitual abortion except in the very specific syndrome of inadequate luteal phase.

SPECIAL CONSIDERATIONS IN PREGNANCY

The effectiveness of progestins in preventing premature delivery remains controversial. Their use in preventing abortion (other than in the case of inadequate luteal phase) is unproved.

At least one random prospective double-blind study has investigated the benefits of administering 17-hydroxyprogesterone caproate prophylactically to a group of women with histories of prior premature deliveries. The group receiving this hormone exhibited a significantly lower prematurity rate than did placebo-treated controls. The rationale for this therapy is based upon the hypothesis that labor is at least partially a result of low or falling progesterone levels.

The use of natural progestins and their esterified derivatives during pregnancy has been associated with limb anomalies, but the literature is unclear as to whether any causal relationship exists. Uterine levels of progesterone are extremely high during pregnancy, and it is difficult to imagine exogenously administered *natural* progesterones having an effect on the fetus. Much of the skepticism about their efficacy in preventing abortion or premature delivery is based on the relatively small contribution made by the exogenous hormone to very high local tissue levels.

DOSAGE

In the maintenance of pregnancy with a luteal phase defect, the usual recommendation is to give progesterone vaginal suppositories 25 mg bid until the twelfth week, or progesterone in oil, 150 mg IM every other day until the twelfth week. In the study mentioned above in which 17-hydroxyprogesterone caproate was given to prevent premature labor, the dose was 250 mg IM every week from the eighteenth to thirty-seventh week of gestation.

ADVERSE EFFECTS

Side effects of progesterone include weight gain and occasional episodes of depression. Because plasma progesterone levels are generally quite high in pregnancy, the addition of exogenous hormone should not cause noticeable side effects.

MECHANISM OF ACTION

Naturally occurring progesterone works at the intracellular level to produce many physiological changes, among which is smooth muscle relaxation. This effect on the uterine musculature is probably critical for the maintenance of pregnancy. Exogenously administered progesterone may supplement that produced by the corpus luteum in early pregnancy and is therefore useful in the management of an inadequate luteal phase. In the absence of this condition, the prevailing evidence is that progestins are not useful in preventing first trimester abortion.

ABSORPTION AND BIOTRANSFORMATION

These drugs are generally given parenterally and hydrolyzed in the liver to pregnanediol and pregnanediol derivatives that are excreted in the urine. Natural progesterone can be absorbed vaginally from suppositories. The progestins are secreted in breast milk at a concentration of 1% to 10% of their blood levels.

Synthetic 19 Nortestosterone Derivatives

INDICATIONS AND RECOMMENDATIONS

Progestins derived from 19 nortestosterone are contraindicated during pregnancy. They are used as oral contraceptive agents and as pregnancy tests. These compounds have also been utilized in attempts to prevent abortion or premature delivery, or both. They are contraindicated because of reported associations between their use and cardiac anomalies, limb reduction defects, and masculinization of the female fetus. If progestin therapy is felt to be necessary during pregnancy, natural progesterone and its esters may be associated with less risk to the fetus.

If they are taken inadvertently during the first trimester, the patient should be told of the potential adverse sequelae. Although incidence figures are not available, the risk to the fetus appears to be small and elective termination of the pregnancy does not seem to be warranted.

RECOMMENDED READING

Aarskog, D. Maternal progestins as a possible cause of hypospadias. *N. Engl. J. Med.* 300:75–78, 1979.

Chez, R. A. Proceedings of the symposium Progesterone, Progestins, and Fetal Development. *Fertil. Steril.* 30:16–26, 1978.

Hill, L. M., Johnson, C. E., and Lee, R. A. Prophylactic use of hydroxy-progesterone caproate in abdominal surgery during pregnancy. *Obstet. Gynecol.* 46:287–290, 1975.

Johnson, J. W. C., Austin, K. L., Jones, G. S., Davis, G. H., and King, T. N. Efficacy of 17 alpha-hydroxyprogesterone caproate in the prevention of premature labor. *N. Engl. J. Med.* 293:675–680, 1975.

Keith, L., and Berger, G. S. The relationship between congenital defects and the use of exogenous progestational "contraceptive" hormones during pregnancy: A 20-year review. *Int. J. Gynecol. Obstet.* 15:115–124, 1977.

Nora, J. J., Nora, A. H., Blu, J., Ingram, J., Fountain, A., Peterson, M., Lortsher, R. H., and Kimberling, W. J. Exogenous progestogen and estrogen implicated in birth defects. *J.A.M.A.* 240:837–843, 1978.

(AHD)

Propranolol (Inderal®)

INDICATIONS AND RECOMMENDATIONS

The use of propranolol during pregnancy should be limited to the treatment of specific life-threatening conditions. These include therapy of thyroid storm, reduction of afterload on the heart in patients at risk to dissect an aortic aneurysm, control of beta-adrenergic side effects of intravenous hydralazine therapy for an acute hypertensive episode, idiopathic hypertrophic subaortic stenosis, and any other life-threatening condition for which there is no acceptable alternative to beta-adrenergic blockade.

When propranolol is given to a pregnant patient for long-term therapy, the fetus must be closely followed for evidence of intrauterine growth retardation. When propranolol is administered during labor, both mother and fetus should have continuous cardiac monitoring, especially if general anesthesia is used.

Newborn infants of mothers who received long-term propranolol during pregnancy should be carefully observed for bradycardia and disturbances of carbohydrate metabolism.

SPECIAL CONSIDERATIONS IN PREGNANCY

Intravenous administration during dysfunctional labor has been reported to increase coordinated contraction patterns without an appreciable concomitant elevation in resting tonus. More experimental work in this setting is needed, however, before the use of propranolol for the treatment of dysfunctional labor can be recommended.

Experiments with pregnant sheep have demonstrated a significant reduction in umbilical flow when propranolol was given intravenously to the mother.

Propranolol easily crosses the placenta and is also secreted into breast milk. Long-term administration of this drug to pregnant women has been associated with growth retardation of the fetus, neonatal hypoglycemia, and bradycardia persisting through the first day of life. In addition, neonates of mothers given intravenous propranolol immediately prior to cesarean section have had difficulty in establishing spontaneous respiratory activity. Propranolol appears in breast milk in amounts that are probably too small to affect the nursing infant.

DOSAGE

When given orally, propranolol appears in the plasma within 30 minutes, and peak levels are obtained 60–90 minutes after administration. When given as a single dose, the half-life is 2–3 hours, but this is increased to 3½–6 hours when the drug is administered over a long period of time. The usual oral doses range from 10–100 mg every 6 hours.

Intravenous doses are given slowly, 1 mg at a time, with a range of from 1 to 5 mg. Careful cardiac monitoring is necessary during intravenous administration.

ADVERSE EFFECTS

Numerous side effects may occur with the use of propranolol. These include sinus bradycardia in most patients and congestive heart failure in those with poor cardiac reserve who cannot tolerate a reduction in cardiac output. Bronchospasm occurs in 2%–10% of patients, and a history of asthma is a contraindication to the use of propranolol. Compromised peripheral circulation may be worsened, and Raynaud's phenomenon is a contraindication to the drug's use. Central nervous system effects include insomnia, nightmares, hallucinations, depression, paresthesias, ataxia, and dizziness. Hyperglycemia may occur, and acute hypertensive episodes have been reported in patients with pheochromocytoma. Finally, an acute hypertensive episode may ensue if propranolol is given with methyldopa. It is hypothesized that alpha-methylnorepinephrine, a metabolite of methyldopa, becomes a potent pressor agent in the presence of a beta-adrenergic blockade.

MECHANISM OF ACTION

Beta-adrenergic blockade produced by propranolol causes decreased cardiac output, slowing of the heart rate, and prolonged mechanical systole. Propranolol also inhibits the release of renin by the kidney and has a direct action on the central nervous system to lower blood pressure. This drug also blocks the adrenergic signs and symptoms of severe thyrotoxicosis.

Intravenous administration causes a rapid fall in heart rate and cardiac output by directly decreasing the force and frequency of myocardial contractions. Initially there is a rise in peripheral vascular resistance and no change or a slight decrease in blood pressure. An antihypertensive effect begins several hours after administration, especially in patients with elevated plasma renin activity. This occurs because of the persistent decrease in cardiac output as well as a fall in peripheral resistance back to or below control levels. The latter may be due to the central action of the drug or to its inhibition of the release of renal renin.

Respiratory airway resistance is consistently increased because of the lack of beta-adrenergic stimulation. Insulin release is mediated by beta-adrenergic mechanisms, and propranolol may therefore interfere with the normal response to an elevation in blood glucose.

ABSORPTION AND BIOTRANSFORMATION

Propranolol is completely absorbed from the gastrointestinal tract, but much of it is rapidly metabolized by the liver. Its half-life ranges from 3½–6 hours. The major metabolite, 4-hydroxypropranolol, is equipotent with propranolol but has a very short half-life.

Renal insufficiency has very little effect on the metabolism of propranolol, and its dosage regimen need not be changed in patients with compromised renal function.

Phenobarbital increases the clearance and decreases the half-life of the drug so that more propranolol may be needed in patients taking both drugs.

RECOMMENDED READING

Anderson, P. O., and Salter, F. J.   Propranolol therapy during pregnancy and lactation (Letter). *Am. J. Cardiol.* 37:325, 1976.

Frohlich, E. D.   The sympathetic depressant antihypertensives. *Drug Ther.* 5:24–33, 1975.

Gladstone, G. R., Hordof, A., and Gersony, W. M.   Propranolol administration during pregnancy: Effects on the fetus. *J. Pediatr.* 86:962–964, 1975.

Holland, O. B., and Kaplan, N. M.   Propranolol in the treatment of hypertension. *N. Engl. J. Med.* 294:930–936, 1976.

Oakes, G. K., Walker, A. M., Ehrenkranz, R. A., and Chez, R. A.   Effect of propranolol infusion on the umbilical and uterine circulations of pregnant sheep. *Am. J. Obstet. Gynecol.* 126:1038–1042, 1976.

Woods, J. R., and Brinkman, C. R., III   The treatment of gestational hypertension. *J. Reprod. Med.* 15:195–199, 1975.

(RLB)

Protamine Sulfate

INDICATIONS AND RECOMMENDATIONS

The use of protamine sulfate during pregnancy should be limited to the treatment of excessive anticoagulation due to an overdose of heparin. In this instance the risk of maternal hemorrhage outweighs consideration of direct toxicity to the fetus.

SPECIAL CONSIDERATIONS IN PREGNANCY

No information is available regarding the safety of this drug in animals or humans during pregnancy.

DOSAGE

Each milligram of protamine sulfate neutralizes approximately 100 mg of heparin. It should be given intravenously at a rate of no more than 50 mg over a 10-minute period. Protamine itself possesses anticoagulant properties and it is therefore unwise to give more than 100 mg over a short period, unless there is certain knowledge of a larger requirement. This will avoid "overneutralization" of the heparin. Because of the rapid clearance of heparin, proportionately less protamine should be administered when more than a half-hour has passed following administration of the former.

ADVERSE EFFECTS

Hypotension, the most common side effect of protamine, is usually associated with infusion at rates greater than 50 mg/10 min. Bradycardia, dyspnea, and transitory flushing may also be associated with rapid infusion. Allergic reactions have been reported following protamine administration to persons allergic to fish.

MECHANISM OF ACTION

The protamines are simple, low-molecular-weight, strongly basic proteins found in the sperm of certain fish. They are able to combine with the strongly acidic heparin and form a stable salt with loss of anticoagulant activity. The protamine-heparin complex is excreted in the kidney.

RECOMMENDED READING

Caplan, S. N., and Berkman, E. M. Protamine sulfate and fish allergy (Letter). *N. Engl. J. Med.* 295:172, 1976.

Goldstein, A., Aronow, L., and Kalman, S. M. *Principles of Drug Action.* New York: Harper & Row, 1968.

Goodman, L. S., and Gilman, A. *The Pharmacological Basis of Therapeutics* (5th ed.). New York: Macmillan, 1975. P. 1354.

(BDH)

Pyrantel Pamoate (Antiminth®)

INDICATIONS AND RECOMMENDATIONS

The use of pyrantel pamoate during pregnancy should be limited to treatment of infections due to susceptible helminths when the mother's well-being is compromised. It is a broad-spectrum antihelminthic agent useful in the treatment of hookworm, roundworm, pinworm, and (investigationally) *Trichostrongylus* infections. Since most parasitic infections are not life-threatening, it is safest to defer therapy until after delivery. Examples of infections that might be treated include a chronic hookworm infection that has produced a significant anemia and heavy roundworm infection with potential for intestinal obstruction.

SPECIAL CONSIDERATIONS IN PREGNANCY

Although teratogenicity has not been described in animals, no human data are available.

DOSAGE

For hookworm (*Ancyclostoma duodenale* or *Necator americanus*), roundworm (*Ascaris lumbricoides*), and *Trichostrongylus* species 11 mg/kg (up to a maximum of 1 gm) is given as a single oral dose. For pinworm (*Enterobius vermicularis*) the same dose is given and repeated in two weeks.

Pyrantel pamoate is supplied as a suspension containing 50 mg of base per milliliter.

ADVERSE EFFECTS

Pyrantel has caused complete neuromuscular blockade in animals given the drug parenterally. Oral doses in humans are relatively free of side effects, with the exception of occasional gastrointestinal disturbance, headache, dizziness, rash, or fever.

MECHANISM OF ACTION

Pyrantel is a depolarizing neuromuscular blocking agent that paralyzes the worm, allowing it to be eliminated in the feces. Pyrantel pamoate is a thousand times more effective than piperazine, a hyperpolarizing agent, for *A. lumbricoides* infections. Pyrantel and piperazine are mutually antagonistic.

ABSORPTION AND BIOTRANSFORMATION

The drug is poorly absorbed from the gastrointestinal tract with less than 15% of the parent compound or its metabolites recovered in the urine.

RECOMMENDED READING

Drugs for parasitic infections. *Med. Lett. Drugs Ther.* 24:17–24, 1978.
Goodman, L. S., and Gilman, A. *The Pharmacological Basis of Therapeutics* (5th ed.). New York: Macmillan, 1975. P. 1028.

LaPorte, V. D., and Gibbs, R. S.   Acute pancreatitis in pregnancy with *Ascaris* infestation. *Obstet. Gynecol.* 49(Suppl 1):84S–85S, 1977.

Pitts, N. E., and Migliardi, J. R.   Antiminth (pyrantel pamoate). *Clin. Pediatr.* (Phila.) 13:87–94, 1974.

(TKH)

Quinidine (Cardioquin®, Quinaglute®)

INDICATIONS AND RECOMMENDATIONS

Quinidine is safe to use during pregnancy. It is an antiarrhythmic used in both atrial and ventricular arrhythmias. It may be administered to pregnant women if it is felt to be the drug of choice for the particular arrhythmia encountered.

SPECIAL CONSIDERATIONS IN PREGNANCY

Although quinine, a compound related to quinidine, appears to have oxytocic properties and is reported to be an abortifacient, the oxytocic properties of quinidine itself are considered to be insignificant.

Quinidine has been shown to cross the placenta, with levels in the fetus being slightly lower than those in the mother. Neonatal thrombocytopenia has been reported. Although eighth-nerve damage has also been reported, it was associated with much higher doses than are ordinarily used.

DOSAGE

The usual maintenance dosage of quinidine sulfate or quinidine gluconate is 200–300 mg PO every 6 hours. Serum levels should be monitored, the therapeutic range being 3–6 μg/ml. Intravenous administration of quinidine should only be undertaken in hospitalized patients who can have continuous electrocardiographic monitoring.

ADVERSE EFFECTS

The most common toxic effects of quinidine are gastrointestinal. Cardiac effects include acceleration of existing atrial arrhythmias and ventricular tachycardia. Idiosyncratic reactions, such as angioedema and vascular collapse, may occur more commonly than with many other drugs.

MECHANISM OF ACTION

Quinidine increases the threshold for electrical excitation and decreases the conduction velocity in cardiac tissue. Other actions include an increase in the effective refractory period, and vagal blockade. Quinidine therapy is effective in the prevention or abolition of such cardiac arrhythmias as atrial fibrillation, atrial flutter, paroxysmal supraventricular and ventricular tachycardia, and premature systoles.

ABSORPTION AND BIOTRANSFORMATION

Quinidine salts are nearly completely absorbed after oral administration, with maximal effects occurring in 1 to 3 hours. Quinidine is metabolized in the liver, primarily to 2-hydroxy-quinidine. Ten to fifty percent of the administered drug is excreted unchanged in the urine within 24 hours.

RECOMMENDED READING

Aviado, D. M., and Salem, H. Drug action, reaction and interaction: I. Quinidine for cardiac arrhythmias. *J. Clin. Pharmacol.* 15:477–485, 1975.

Goodman, L. S., and Gilman, A. *The Pharmacological Basis of Therapeutics* (5th ed.). New York: Macmillan, 1975. Pp. 686–694.

Hill, L. M., and Malkasian, G. D. The use of quinidine sulfate throughout pregnancy. *Obstet. Gynecol.* 54:366–368, 1979.

(MJM)

Quinine

INDICATIONS AND RECOMMENDATIONS

The use of quinine during pregnancy should be limited to the treatment of attacks of chloroquine-resistant falciparum malaria. In this particular situation, the risk of teratogenicity is outweighed by that of congenital malaria. Its use is not warranted in the treatment of nocturnal leg cramps in light of its oxytocic and possible teratogenic effects.

SPECIAL CONSIDERATIONS IN PREGNANCY

Quinine is known to have an oxytocic action in the pregnant woman. The nongravid human uterus is only slightly influenced, but as pregnancy proceeds the oxytocic action of quinine becomes more noticeable. Toxic amounts of the drug may cause abortion.

Quinine crosses the placental barrier and causes toxicity in the fetus. Congenital anomalies of the eye and deafness have been attributed to quinine use during pregnancy.

DOSAGE

The dose of quinine given in the treatment of uncomplicated attacks of falciparum malaria is 650 mg tid for 10–14 days. It should be given in conjunction with pyrimethamine, sulfadiazine, or (in the nonpregnant patient) tetracycline.

ADVERSE EFFECTS

Therapeutic doses of quinine can produce cinchonism, a syndrome that includes tinnitus, headache, nausea, and visual disturbances. With continued treatment or large doses, dermatological, gastrointestinal, central nervous system, and cardiovascular symptoms may become prominent. Hematological side effects are rare and include hemolytic anemia; hypoprothrombinemia, which can be reversed by vitamin K; and thrombocytopenia.

MECHANISM OF ACTION

Quinine has been described as a "general protoplasmic poison" affecting many enzyme systems. Its exact mechanism as an antimalarial is unknown. It has activity as an analgesic and is a poor antipyretic. It exhibits cardiovascular effects similar to its isomer quinidine, oxytocic activity in late pregnancy, and curare-like effects on skeletal muscle.

ABSORPTION AND BIOTRANSFORMATION

Quinine is readily absorbed from the gastrointestinal tract. Peak levels are seen 1–3 hours after an oral dose. Approximately 70% of plasma quinine is bound to proteins. It is cleared primarily by the liver with less than 5% of the dose excreted unchanged in the urine.

RECOMMENDED READING

Drugs for parasitic infections. *Med. Lett. Drugs Ther.* 20:17–24, 1978.

Goodman, L. S., and Gilman, A. *The Pharmacological Basis of Therapeutics* (5th ed.). New York: Macmillan, 1975. Pp. 1062–1065.

Heinonen, O. P., Slone, O., and Shapiro, S. (Eds.). *Birth Defects and Drugs in Pregnancy.* Littleton, Mass.: Publishing Sciences Group, 1977. Pp. 299–302, 313.

Lewis, R., Lauerson, N. H., and Birnbaum, S. Malaria associated with pregnancy. *Obstet. Gynecol.* 42:696–700, 1973.

Siroty, R. R.   Purpura on the rocks—with a twist. *J.A.M.A.* 235:2521–2522, 1976.

Sutherland, J. M., and Light, I. J.   The effect of drugs upon the fetus. *Pediatr. Clin. North Am.* 12:781–806, 1965.

(TKH)

Rauwolfia Alkaloids: Reserpine (Sandril®, Serpasil®, Raurine®)

INDICATIONS AND RECOMMENDATIONS

The rauwolfia alkaloids are relatively contraindicated during pregnancy because other therapeutic agents are preferable. Reserpine is one of approximately twenty related compounds that comprise this family of antihypertensive agents. They act by depleting the natural stores of biogenic amines in the brain, myocardium, adrenal medulla, and postganglionic nerve endings. The transport of norepinephrine into its storage granules is blocked and the reuptake of released catecholamines by the nerve endings is inhibited. The hypotensive action of these drugs is due to a reduction in sympathetic stimulation of the blood vessels and heart and is associated with a bradycardia as well as a decrease in vascular resistance.

Side effects include postural and exercise hypotension, although these are uncommon when the drug is taken orally in effective amounts. Unopposed parasympathetic stimulation may cause an increase in gastric acid secretion, peptic ulceration, frequent bowel movements or diarrhea, prolonged atrioventricular conduction, and enhanced second-degree heart block. Nasal arteriolar dilation may result in nasal stuffiness. Brain amine and serotonin depletion can cause depression and behavioral changes, and these serve as limiting factors in the long-term administration of high enough doses to cause major sympathoplegia. Some epidemiological studies suggest an association of reserpine therapy with breast cancer.

Reserpine crosses the placenta, and the major fetal complication is neonatal respiratory difficulty secondary to nasal congestion. Reserpine also appears in the breast milk. Although no case reports have been published, the same risks may exist for nursing infants as for neonates exposed in utero.

Although some authors recommend reserpine as an alternative drug in the therapy of chronic hypertension during pregnancy, the large number of maternal side effects make this a less attractive choice than other agents that are currently available.

RECOMMENDED READING

Armstrong, B., Stevens, N., and Doll, R.   Retrospective study of the association between use of rauwolfia derivatives and breast cancer in English women. *Lancet* 2:672–675, 1974.
Goodman, L. S., and Gilman, A.   *The Pharmacological Basis of Therapeutics* (5th ed.). New York: Macmillan, 1975. Pp. 557–559.
Lee, P. A., Kelly, M. R., and Wallin, J. D.   Increased prolactin levels during reserpine treatment of hypertensive patients. *J.A.M.A.* 235:2316–2317, 1976.
Reserpine. *Med. Lett. Drugs Ther.* 18:19–20, 1976.

(RLB)

Ritodrine (Yutopar®)

INDICATIONS AND RECOMMENDATIONS

Ritodrine is the first and only beta adrenergic drug approved by the Food and Drug Administration (FDA) for use as a tocolytic agent. It is a beta-2 adrenergic agonist which primarily acts upon myometrial receptors.

Ritodrine's major usefulness is in the treatment of premature labor that is not due to an obvious cause. Premature labor accompanied by chorioamnionitis, fetal death, severe preeclampsia, life-threatening maternal complications, or severe third-trimester bleeding should be allowed to continue, and is thus a contraindication to the use of a tocolytic agent. Women with cardiac disease may be adversely affected by the cardiovascular effects of ritodrine and diabetic control may be compromised by its effects on carbohydrate metabolism. Finally, great care must be exercised when ritodrine is used in combination with glucocorticoids, because of the possibility of causing pulmonary edema.

SPECIAL CONSIDERATIONS IN PREGNANCY

Ritodrine decreases the intensity and frequency of uterine contractions in women with spontaneous or induced labor. It has been found to be more effective than either placebo or ethanol. Prospective clinical trials comparing ritodrine with other selective beta-2 agonists are necessary in order to assess their relative effectiveness as tocolytic agents. The incidence of maternal cardiovascular side effects with ritodrine is reported to be lower than with less selective beta-2 agonists such as isoxsuprine.

Ritodrine is not indicated for use in the first half of pregnancy. Nevertheless, to date there are no reports of teratogenesis in humans associated with the use of this drug during embryogenesis. Ritodrine crosses the placenta but cord concentrations are lower than concomitant maternal values.

Uterine and placental blood flow are increased in women taking this drug and fetal tachycardia may occur following maternal administration. It has also been shown to increase maternal and fetal serum glucose concentrations, as well as maternal insulin levels. Because neonatal hypoglycemia has been observed with maternal administration of other beta-2 adrenergic agonists, infants who were exposed to ritodrine in utero should be carefully followed for this problem. Diabetic mothers taking this drug may need increased doses of insulin in order to maintain adequate glucose control.

Ritodrine has been used outside of the United States in the treatment of acute intrapartum fetal distress. It has not been approved for this use in the United States. The role of ritodrine in the prophylaxis of premature labor in multiple pregnancy requires further study.

No data exist concerning the secretion of ritodrine in breast milk, but since it is not indicated for use after delivery and the half-life is quite short, it is unlikely that ritodrine would cause significant problems in the nursing infant.

DOSAGE

Ritodrine is administered intravenously by constant infusion. The recommended starting dose is 100 μg/min. This should be increased in 50 μg/min increments every 10 minutes until a dose which provides satisfactory tocolytic action has been reached. Maternal cardiovascular side effects may be a limiting factor. The maximal recommended infusion rate is 350 μg/min.

The intravenous infusion is maintained until satisfactory tocolysis has been achieved. Thirty minutes prior to termination of the intravenous infusion, oral ritodrine is begun. Oral dosage is 10 mg every 2 hours. The initial oral dose is maintained for 24 hours and then reduced, if possible, to 10–20 mg every 4–6 hours. Generally, oral therapy is continued until the pregnancy has reached term. Intramuscular ritodrine is not available for use in this country.

ADVERSE EFFECTS

The most frequent side effects of ritodrine are cardiovascular. Maternal tachycardia may occur due to its chronotropic activity. Occasionally premature ventricular contractions are seen. Ritodrine also increases stroke volume and, therefore, systolic pressure. Peripheral vascular resistance, on the other hand, is decreased and this reduces diastolic pressure and consequently widens the pulse pressure.

Ritodrine may cause hyperglycemia which can lead to metabolic acidosis in poorly controlled diabetic women. In addition, an incompletely understood form of metabolic acidosis accompanied by an increased anion gap has been reported in association with mild hyperglycemia.

Pulmonary edema has been reported with the combined use of glucocorticoids and other beta adrenergic agonists. Although, thus far, this problem has not been described with ritodrine, it should be anticipated. Patients being given ritodrine in combination with steroids should certainly not be fluid-overloaded.

MECHANISM OF ACTION

Ritodrine is a sympathomimetic agent with predominantly beta-2 activity. It is believed that such agents stimulate adenyl cyclase, the enzyme which catalyzes the conversion of ATP to cyclic AMP. Increased intracellular concentrations of cyclic AMP cause relaxation of the uterine musculature.

ABSORPTION AND BIOTRANSFORMATION

Orally administered ritodrine is rapidly absorbed in the gastrointestinal tract. Bioavailability of an oral dose is approximately 30%. The drug is conjugated in the liver, with plasma half-life being 1.3–2 hours. Ninety percent of the drug may be recovered from the urine within 24 hours of administration.

RECOMMENDED READING

Bieniarz, J., Ivankovich, A., and Scommegna, A.   Cardiac output during ritodrine treatment in premature labor. *Am. J. Obstet. Gynecol.* 118:910–920, 1974.

Boog, G., Brahim, M. B., and Gandar, R.   Beta-mimetic drugs and possible prevention of respiratory distress syndrome. *Br. J. Obstet. Gynaecol.* 82:285–288, 1975.

Brettes, J. P., Renand, R., and Gandar, R.   A double-blind investigation into the effects of ritodrine on uterine blood flow during the third trimester of pregnancy. *Am. J. Obstet. Gynecol.* 124:164–168, 1976.

Humphrey, M., Chang, A., Gilbert, M., and Wood, C.   The effect of intra-venous ritodrine on the acid-base status of the fetus during the second stage of labor. *Br. J. Obstet. Gynaecol.* 82:234–245, 1975.

Landesman, R., Wilson, K. H., Coutinho, E., Klima, I. M., and Marcus, R. S.   The relaxant action of ritodrine, a sympathomimetic amine, on the uterus during term labor. *Am. J. Obstet. Gynecol.* 110:111–114, 1971.

Laurersen, N. H., Maerkatz, I. R., Tejani, N., Wilson, K. H., Roberson, A., Mann, L. I., and Luchs, F.   Inhibition of premature labor: A multicentric comparison of ritodrine and ethanol. *Am. J. Obstet. Gynecol.* 127:836–845, 1977.

Nochimscn, D. J., Riffel, H. D., Yeh, S., Kreitzer, M. S., Paul, R. H., and Hon, E. H.   The effects of ritodrine hydrochloride on uterine activity and the cardiovascular system. *Am. J. Obstet. Gynecol.* 118:523–528, 1974.

Wesselius-DeCasparis, A., Thiery, M., Yolesian, A., Baumgarten, K., Bros-fins, I., Gamissan, O., Stolk, J. G., and Vivier, W.   Results of a double-blind, multicentric study with ritodrine in premature labor. *Br. Med. J.* 3:144–147, 1971.

(RJR)

Salicylates: Sodium salicylate, Acetylsalicyclic acid (Aspirin)

INDICATIONS AND RECOMMENDATIONS

The use of salicylates in pregnancy should be limited to their employment as anti-inflammatory agents in the treatment of various forms of arthritis. They should be considered as second-line analgesic and antipyretic drugs, since acetaminophen is an effective agent for such use with less potential for toxicity. If patients are sensitive to acetaminophen, however, salicylates may be administered.

Because of possible fetal sequelae it is not judicious to utilize salicylates for their antiplatelet aggregation effect. Should anticoagulation be needed, heparin is the agent of choice. Long-term salicylate therapy may be necessary for treating arthritis during pregnancy; if so, prothrombin time and hemoglobin levels should be monitored closely.

Patients taking large doses of salicylates during pregnancy may have prolonged gestations. Any patient on such therapy whose pregnancy exceeds 42 weeks from her last menstrual period should be followed closely to rule out the postmaturity syndrome.

SPECIAL CONSIDERATIONS IN PREGNANCY

Prolongation of the bleeding time can occur with one 325-mg aspirin tablet, while 650 mg, the usual dose, has been shown to double the mean bleeding time for 4–7 days. Although this would be of most concern in the third trimester, spontaneous abortion, premature labor, and placental hemorrhage make bleeding diatheses a potential problem at any time during pregnancy. Increased length of gestation and a longer labor have been described in long-term salicylate users, presumably due to an antiprostaglandin effect.

Potential fetal problems include increased bleeding time and jaundice (due to competition with bilirubin for albumin binding). The incidence of cephalhematoma and melena is reportedly increased in neonates exposed to salicylates in utero. Various severe birth defects have been anecdotally reported in the offspring of salicylate users, but no cause-and-effect relationship has been established. Premature closure of the ductus arteriosus is a theoretical risk of salicylate ingestion because of its antiprostaglandin action. This may be responsible for the slightly increased perinatal mortality reported among salicylate users.

DOSAGE

The usual analgesic/antipyretic dose for aspirin or sodium salicylate is 162–650 mg every 4 hours. Higher doses are often used for severe arthritis.

ADVERSE EFFECTS

Side effects of acetylsalicylic acid are numerous; these include gastrointestinal irritation and bleeding, pylorospasm and vomiting, increased bile flow, and increased bleeding due to inhibition of platelet function. Iron deficiency anemia may occur with long-term use. Toxic doses of salicylates may precipitate fatty liver, renal damage, and central nervous system disturbances (including restlessness, incoherent speech, tremor, delirium, and even convulsions, coma, and toxic encephalopathy). Initial hyperventilation may lead to respiratory alkalosis, but increased oxygen consumption and renal damage may eventually produce a metabolic acidosis.

MECHANISM OF ACTION

Salicylates act peripherally by inhibiting prostaglandin synthesis in inflamed tissues. This prevents the sensitization of pain receptors to mechanical or chemical stimulation. They inhibit histamine release, render neutrophils unresponsive to chemotactic stimuli, and interfere with granulocyte adherence. At high dosage, as used for the therapy of arthritis, they interfere with formation of antigen-antibody complexes and suppress lymphocyte function. The antipyretic action of salicylates is mediated via hypothalamic centers and may be due to inhibition of prostaglandin E release. Because acetylsalicylic acid preparations reduce platelet aggregation by inhibiting the release of platelet adenosine diphosphate (ADP), they are sometimes prescribed as mild anticoagulants.

Physiological effects include relief of low intensity pain, antipyresis, anti-inflammatory action, reduction in fatty acid and cholesterol concentration, increased urinary excretion of urates, and decreased platelet aggregation.

ABSORPTION AND BIOTRANSFORMATION

Sodium salicylate and acetylsalicylic acid are the most commonly available forms of this compound. Oral administration leads to rapid absorption, with therapeutic effects observed 20–30 minutes after ingestion. Salicylates are absorbed in the stomach and upper small intestine. Although absorption is fastest at low pH, solubility increases with rising pH such that "buffering" agents have little effect on absorption. Rectal absorption is unreliable.

The absorbed drug is distributed to all tissues of the body, including cerebrospinal fluid. Fifty to ninety percent of salicylates is bound to serum albumin. Excretion is mainly renal and increases with alkalinization of the urine. The apparent half-life of salicylates is dependent upon the serum concentration and ranges from 3–22 hours.

RECOMMENDED READING

Collins, E., and Turner, C. Aspirin during pregnancy (Letter). *Lancet* 2:797–798, 1976.

Collins, E., and Turner, C. Maternal effects of regular salicylate ingestion in pregnancy. *Lancet* 2:335–339, 1975.

Goodman, L. S., and Gilman, A. *The Pharmacological Basis of Therapeutics* (5th ed.). New York: Macmillan, 1975. Pp. 325–339.

Jamieson, D., and Buckle, P. A comparison of anti-inflammatory and other compounds on the spontaneously contracting pregnant rat uterus. *J. Pharm. Pharmacol.* 29:112–114, 1977.

Roe, R. L. Drug therapy in rheumatic diseases. *Med. Clin. North Am.* 61:405–418, 1977.

(BRS)

Scopolamine

INDICATIONS AND RECOMMENDATIONS

Scopolamine is contraindicated during pregnancy. This drug is an anticholinergic agent used as a preanesthetic to decrease salivary secretions and produce amnesia. When used antepartum, it causes depression of the neonate. Since much more effective anesthetic adjuncts are available, the use of this drug during pregnancy is not recommended.

The use of scopolamine in over-the-counter medications is discussed under *Belladonna alkaloids*.

RECOMMENDED READING

Goodman, L. S., and Gilman, A. *The Pharmacological Basis of Therapeutics* (5th ed.). New York: Macmillan, 1975. Pp. 515–523.
McDonald, J. S. Preanesthetic and intrapartal medications. *Clin. Obstet. Gynecol.* 20:447–459, 1977.

(PCL)

Simethicone (over-the-counter)
(Mylicon®, Silain®)

INDICATIONS AND RECOMMENDATIONS

Simethicone is safe to use during pregnancy. It is used for the relief of gaseous distention, bloating, or flatulence.

SPECIAL CONSIDERATIONS IN PREGNANCY

There are no special considerations related to pregnancy.

DOSAGE

The usual dose is 40–80 mg chewed thoroughly three to four times a day.

ADVERSE EFFECTS

There are no known side effects.

MECHANISM OF ACTION

Simethicone is a mixture of silica gel and dimethylpolysiloxanes. Their defoaming action relieves flatulence by dispersing and preventing the formation of mucus-surrounded gas pockets in the gastrointestinal tract. Simethicone changes the surface tension of gas bubbles in the stomach and intestine, allowing them to coalesce. The gas is freed and is eliminated easily by belching or passing flatus.

ABSORPTION AND BIOTRANSFORMATION

It is not absorbed to any extent.

RECOMMENDED READING

Goodman, L. S., and Gilman, A. *The Pharmacological Basis of Therapeutics* (5th ed.). New York: Macmillan, 1975. P. 949.
Schenkel, B., and Vorherr, H. Non-prescription drugs during pregnancy: Potential teratogenic and toxic effects upon embryo and fetus. *J. Reprod. Med.* 12:27–45, 1974.

(RAC)

Sodium Nitroprusside (Nipride®)

INDICATIONS AND RECOMMENDATIONS

The use of sodium nitroprusside during pregnancy is controversial. It is the most potent and predictably effective drug available for hypertensive emergencies, but it has not been studied enough to define its safety prior to delivery. Animal data are worrisome because they suggest that cyanide toxicity could occur in the fetus while the mother remains asymptomatic. If used at all, sodium nitroprusside should be restricted to the treatment of an acute hypertensive emergency unresponsive to intravenous hydralazine or diazoxide therapy; nitroprusside should only be used to control the acute crisis, and delivery of the infant should be performed as quickly as possible thereafter.

SPECIAL CONSIDERATIONS IN PREGNANCY

No changes in umbilical or uterine blood flow have been observed in pregnant sheep when nitroprusside has been administered. In experiments with pregnant ewes, the administration of steadily increasing doses of nitroprusside given to maintain a 20% reduction in mean arterial pressure was associated with marked accumulation of cyanide in the fetus. Cyanide levels in the fetus were significantly higher than those in the mother and were associated with death in utero. The placenta has therefore been shown to be readily permeable to the nitroprusside molecule and, at least in the sheep model, cyanide trapping seems to occur.

DOSAGE

Nitroprusside is light-sensitive and must be delivered in a system wrapped in a light-shielding material such as aluminum foil. It must be given by infusion pump while the patient's blood pressure is constantly monitored. Because its action is so evanescent, hypertension will recur almost immediately after the infusion is discontinued.

The dosage is variable and must be titrated against the individual patient's requirements. The dosage range is 0.5–8 μg/kg/min by constant IV infusion. The average dose required to sustain a 30%–40% decrease in diastolic pressure is 3 μg/kg/min. The onset is immediate and the duration of action is only as long as the infusion runs.

ADVERSE EFFECTS

Side effects are usually minimal, but prolonged administration can result in cyanide or thiocyanate toxicity. Cyanide is liberated by direct combination of nitroprusside with sulfhydryl groups in red blood cells and tissue. Circulating cyanide is converted to thiocyanate in the liver. Principal manifestations of toxicity are fatigue, nausea, and anorexia followed by disorientation, psychotic behavior, and muscle spasm. Hypothyroidism has been reported following prolonged therapy.

MECHANISM OF ACTION

This drug acts specifically on vascular smooth muscle. Its action is virtually immediate and very evanescent. It therefore must be given through a carefully monitored intravenous infusion.

Nitroprusside causes variable effects on cardiac output and heart rate. These are related to the preexisting state of cardiac performance and are secondary to reductions in peripheral resistance and venous tone. There are no demonstrable effects on the autonomic or central nervous systems.

ABSORPTION AND BIOTRANSFORMATION

Nitroprusside is metabolized to thiocyanate, which is excreted almost exclusively by the kidney. Its half-life is approximately 1 week in patients with normal renal function.

RECOMMENDED READING

Kelly, J. V.   Drugs used in the management of toxemia of pregnancy. *Clin. Obstet. Gynecol.* 20:395–410, 1977.

Lewis, P. E., Cefalo, R. C., Naulty, J. S., and Rodkey, F. L.   Placental transfer and fetal toxicity of sodium nitroprusside. *Gynecol. Invest.* 8:46–47, 1977.

Palmer, R. F., and Lasseter, K. C.   Drug therapy: Sodium nitroprusside. *N. Engl. J. Med.* 292:294–297, 1975.

(RLB)

Spironolactone (Aldactone®)

INDICATIONS AND RECOMMENDATIONS

Spironolactone is relatively contraindicated during pregnancy. If diuretics are necessary at that time the thiazides or furosemide are preferable. Serum potassium levels should be followed closely whenever pregnant women are given diuretics. If hypokalemia develops with the thiazide diuretics, oral potassium supplementation will effectively correct this problem. There is therefore no important advantage of spironolactone over these other agents, the effects of which in pregnancy are better known.

Spironolactone is a competitive antagonist of aldosterone for receptor sites in the distal renal tubules. Aldosterone normally acts to augment renal tubular reabsorption of sodium and chloride and to increase the excretion of potassium.

The effects of this drug on uterine blood flow and the fetus have not been well studied. Metabolic products may appear in breast milk.

RECOMMENDED READING

Gifford, R. W., Jr.   A guide to the practical use of diuretics. *J.A.M.A.* 235:1890–1893, 1976.

Goodman, L. S., and Gilman, A.   *The Pharmacological Basis of Therapeutics* (5th ed.). New York: Macmillan, 1975. Pp. 837–838.

(PCL)

Sulfonamides: Sulfadiazine, Sulfamethizole (Thiosulfil Forte®), Sulfamethoxazole (Gantanol®), Sulfisoxazole (Gantrisin®)

INDICATIONS AND RECOMMENDATIONS

Sulfonamides are contraindicated during the last 3 months of pregnancy but may be administered earlier in pregnancy to treat urinary tract infections. These agents are antibiotics with a wide range of activity against both gram-positive and gram-negative organisms. They should not be used during the last 3 months of pregnancy because of the danger of kernicterus to the neonate. If premature delivery is anticipated, these agents should not be administered at any time during the third trimester.

SPECIAL CONSIDERATIONS IN PREGNANCY

There are no unusual maternal effects of sulfonamides during pregnancy. These drugs rapidly cross the placenta and appear in amniotic fluid at a slower rate than in fetal blood. They compete with bilirubin for binding with albumin. In utero the fetus can clear free bilirubin through the placental circulation, but in the neonatal period this route of clearance no longer exists. In the neonate elevated levels of free bilirubin traverse the blood-brain barrier where binding to the basal ganglia, with subsequent kernicterus, may occur.

Sulfonamides appear in breast milk. Infants with glucose 6-phosphate dehydrogenase (G6PD) deficiency might develop hemolytic anemia if nursed by mothers taking sulfonamides. Theoretically, the chance of kernicterus might also be increased in babies with an Rh or ABO incompatibility.

DOSAGE

Table 12 details recommended dosages.

ADVERSE EFFECTS

Frequent side effects consist of allergic reactions that include rash, photosensitivity, and drug fever. Rarely, these drugs can cause hepatic damage; vasculitis; hemolytic anemia, especially in those with G6PD deficiency; and other blood dyscrasias. The long-acting sulfonamides may be associated with the Stevens-Johnson syndrome and can increase the effects of oral anticoagulants. Renal damage may occur as a result of crystalluria, the risk of which, however, may be diminished by maintaining a high urine output.

MECHANISM OF ACTION

The relative antibacterial differences in this group are insignificant, and preferences for one agent over another are based on pharmacological or toxicological considerations. They compete with the para-aminobenzoic acid utilized by bacteria for the synthesis

Table 12. Dosage Chart for Sulfonamides

Drug	Oral Dosage (gm)	Oral Interval (hours)	Usual Maximum Dose/Day (gm)	Dosage Interval for Creatinine Clearance (ml/min) 80–50	Dosage Interval for Creatinine Clearance (ml/min) 50–10	Dosage Interval for Creatinine Clearance (ml/min) Less than 10
Sulfadiazine	0.5–1	q4–6	8	6–8 hours	8–12 hours	12–24 hours
Sulfisoxazole	0.5–1	q4–6	8	6–8 hours	8–12 hours	12–24 hours
Sulfamethizole	0.5–1	q4–6	8	6–8 hours	8–12 hours	12–24 hours
Sulfamethoxazole	1	q8–12	8	(Not recommended)		

of folic acid and act as bacteriostatic agents. They are used primarily to treat urinary tract infections due to susceptible organisms. Other indications for their use include chancroid, trachoma, inclusion conjunctivitis, and nocardiosis.

ABSORPTION AND BIOTRANSFORMATION

These drugs are rapidly absorbed from the small intestine and stomach. They rapidly bind to albumin and are distributed throughout all the tissues of the body. Ten to forty percent is metabolized by acetylation to the inactive form. Both free and acetylated metabolites are excreted in the urine.

RECOMMENDED READING

Davies, D. M. *Textbook of Adverse Drug Reactions*. Oxford: Oxford University Press, 1977. P. 70.

Handbook of Antimicrobial Therapy. The Medical Letter on Drugs and Therapeutics (Rev. ed.). New Rochelle, N.Y.: The Medical Letter, 1978.

Update: Drugs in breast milk. *Med. Lett. Drugs Ther.* 21:21–24, 1979.

(GRD)

Sulfonylureas: Acetohexamide (Dymelor®), Chlorpropamide (Diabinese®), Tolazamide (Tolinase®), Tolbutamide (Orinase®)

INDICATIONS AND RECOMMENDATIONS

Sulfonylureas are relatively contraindicated during pregnancy because other therapeutic agents are preferable. These drugs are orally administered to lower the blood glucose in mild non-ketosis-prone diabetics.

Some studies have shown an increased perinatal mortality in patients treated with sulfonylureas rather than insulin, while other studies have not borne this out. There is evidence of teratogenicity in laboratory animals given high doses of these compounds.

It is known that tolbutamide crosses the placenta easily, and isolated cases of prolonged neonatal hypoglycemia have been reported when the mother was taking this drug. On the other hand, Pederson has used oral agents in a limited number of pregnant patients and reports no unusual hypoglycemia. He does not, however, recommend their use during pregnancy.

It is recommended that the sulfonylureas not be used during pregnancy because of the relative lack of data regarding their safety and efficacy. When diabetes is present during pregnancy, insulin is the drug of choice.

RECOMMENDED READING

Adam, P. A. J., and Schwartz, R. Diagnosis and treatment: Should oral hypoglycemic agents be used in pediatric and pregnant patients? *Pediatrics* 42:819–823, 1968.

Douglas, C. P., and Richards, R. Use of chlorpropamide in the treatment of diabetes in pregnancy. *Diabetes* 16:60–61, 1967.

Jackson, W. P. U., Campbell, G. D., Nobelovitz, M., and Blumsohn, D. Tolbutamide and chlorpropamide during pregnancy in human diabetics. *Diabetes* 11(Suppl):98–101, 1962.

Marble, A., White, P., Bradley, R. F., and Korall, L. P. (Eds.). *Joslin's Diabetes Mellitus* (11th ed.). Philadelphia: Lea & Febiger, 1971.

Pederson, J. *The Pregnant Diabetic and Her Newborn* (2nd ed.). Baltimore: Williams & Wilkins, 1977. Pp. 65–67.

Shen, S. W., and Bressler, R. Clinical pharmacology of oral anti-diabetic agents (Part II of 2 parts). *N. Engl. J. Med.* 296:787–793, 1977.

Sutherland, H. W., Stowers, J. M., Cormack, J. D., and Bewsher, P. D. Evaluation of chlorpropamide in chemical diabetes diagnosed during pregnancy. *Br. Med. J.* 3:9–13, 1973.

(DRC)

Sympathomimetics (over-the-counter): Ephedrine, Phenylephrine, Phenylpropanolamine

INDICATIONS AND RECOMMENDATIONS

Sympathomimetics are generally safe to use during pregnancy, although they should be avoided in patients with essential hypertension or toxemia because of their potential for elevating systemic blood pressure. They should also be avoided in situations in which there is poor fetal reserve, as distress in utero could be precipitated. Members of this group of drugs are used in expectorants, decongestants, cough and cold medications, antiasthmatic combinations, and ophthalmic decongestants and vasoconstrictors.

SPECIAL CONSIDERATIONS IN PREGNANCY

There are no maternal side effects unique to pregnancy. These substances cross the placental and blood-brain barriers and fetal central nervous system effects may include hyperactivity and irritability following maternal ingestion. The fetus may also develop a tachycardia. Maternal hypertension could stress a compromised fetus. Congenital anomalies have not been associated with the use of sympathomimetics in over-the-counter (OTC) preparations.

DOSAGE

The dosage varies with the preparation being used. This group of drugs is most effective when administered orally. Their onset of action is rapid, and they are effective for hours because of their resistance to inactivating enzymes.

ADVERSE EFFECTS

Side effects from these drugs include insomnia, anxiety, headache, tremor, dizziness, palpitations, anorexia, nausea, vomiting, abdominal cramps, and diarrhea.

MECHANISM OF ACTION

The sympathomimetic drugs used in OTC preparations are primarily noncatecholamines. They may act directly on effector cells or act indirectly by stimulating the release of norepinephrine from adrenergic nerve endings. The structure of each substance determines its predominant mode of action.

Ephedrine causes norepinephrine release and has alpha receptor effects. It also has a direct effect on beta receptors in the bronchial tree, resulting in a relaxation of bronchospasm. Phenylephrine acts directly on alpha receptors, especially in the heart. It has little effect on beta receptors, however.

Ephedrine and phenylpropanolamine may cause an increase in systolic and diastolic blood pressures as well as cardiac output. They may also increase alertness, decrease fatigue, and cause mild mood elevation. Phenylephrine can elevate both systolic and diastolic blood pressures and increase circulation time and venous pressure. It may also be associated with a reflex bradycardia.

ABSORPTION AND BIOTRANSFORMATION

The sympathomimetics included in OTC preparations are generally well absorbed from the gastrointestinal tract. Their metabolic pathways include hydroxylation, N-demethylation, deamination, and conjugation in the liver, followed by urinary excretion. They may also be excreted unchanged by the kidneys, the amount depending on urinary pH.

RECOMMENDED READING

Goodman, L. S., and Gilman, A. *The Pharmacological Basis of Therapeutics* (5th ed.). New York: Macmillan, 1975. Pp. 477–511.

Nelson, M. M., and Forfar, J. O. Associations between drugs administered during pregnancy and congenital abnormalities of the fetus. *Br. Med. J.* 1:523–527, 1971.

Schenkel, B., and Vorherr, H. Non-prescription drugs during pregnancy: Potential teratogenic and toxic effects upon embryo and fetus. *J. Reprod. Med.* 12:27–45, 1974.

(RAC)

Terbutaline (Brethine®)

INDICATIONS AND RECOMMENDATIONS

The use of terbutaline during pregnancy should be limited to the treatment of those asthmatic patients who remain symptomatic on maximum doses of theophylline. Patients taking terbutaline orally may concurrently use an aerosol form of another beta-2 adrenergic agent. Concurrent use of other *systemic* beta-2 sympathomimetics should be avoided because of the unpleasant side effects associated with excessive adrenergic stimulation.

Terbutaline has been used to arrest premature labor. At the Yale–New Haven Medical Center it is administered both orally and subcutaneously for this purpose. Although it has not been approved by the Food and Drug Administration (FDA) for this purpose, it has been widely used around the world with significant success and has earned a reputation for relative efficacy and safety.

SPECIAL CONSIDERATIONS IN PREGNANCY

Beta sympathomimetic agents have produced cardiovascular abnormalities in chick embryos. Terbutaline, however, has not been specifically reported to have this effect. There are no published reports of teratogenesis in humans using the drug, although controlled studies establishing its safety during pregnancy are not available.

The effectiveness of terbutaline in inhibiting premature labor has been demonstrated in several clinical trials. One double-blind controlled study found that in 80% of patients premature labor was arrested with terbutaline as compared with 20% in the control group. In addition, this drug has been shown to decrease both spontaneous and oxytocin-stimulated labor at full term. This effect was seen even in the second stage of labor. Terbutaline has been used to treat acute intrapartum fetal distress, but reports are limited in this area.

There is no information regarding the passage of terbutaline across the placenta or into breast milk. For theoretical reasons, however, newborns exposed to terbutaline in utero should be observed for hypoglycemia. An increase in fetal heart rate has been observed following parenteral administration of the drug to pregnant women.

DOSAGE

For treatment of asthma, the oral dose is 2.5–5 mg every 6–8 hours, with onset of action about 30 minutes. Peak effect occurs in 2–3 hours, and the duration of action is usually 4–6 hours. The subcutaneous dose is 0.25 mg, which may be repeated in 30 minutes if no clinical response occurs. If there is no clinical response within the next half hour, other measures should be taken to treat the bronchospasm. The onset of action of subcutaneous terbutaline is about 15 minutes; peak effect occurs in 30–60 minutes; and the duration of action is 1½–4 hours.

Terbutaline aerosols are marketed elsewhere but are not currently available in the United States.

Terbutaline has not been approved by the FDA for the treatment of premature labor. Because of the extensive experience with it in Europe and the United States, the drug is administered for this purpose by the oral and subcutaneous routes at the Yale–New Haven Medical Center. (We have no experience with the intravenous administration of terbutaline and consequently cannot recommend this mode of administration.) The subcutaneous dose is 0.25 mg every 6 hours × 3 days. The treatment regimen is then repeated as often as necessary up to 36 weeks of gestation.

As soon as parenteral terbutaline or any other regimen has arrested premature labor, an oral dose of 2.5–7.5 mg every 6 hours should be given. This regimen is continued up to 36 weeks of gestation.

When given intravenously, the terbutaline dosage is titrated to the patient's needs with a constant infusion. Rates in reported series average about 10 μg/min. The effective rate is maintained for 1 hour after contractions have ceased and then gradually reduced over an 8-hour period. If the procedure is successful, the drug can be given orally as described above.

ADVERSE EFFECTS

Side effects include tachycardia, palpitations, headache, nausea, vomiting, anxiety, sweating, tremor, and tinnitus. With usual doses, side effects are generally transient and do not require treatment.

MECHANISM OF ACTION

Terbutaline is a sympathomimetic agent with predominantly beta-2 activity. It is believed that sympathomimetics work by stimulating adenylcyclase, the enzyme that catalyzes the conversion of adenosine triphosphate to cyclic adenosine monophosphate.

Terbutaline produces significant bronchodilation, which may result in an increased vital capacity, forced expiratory volume in one second (FEV_1), peak expiratory flow (PEF), and maximum expiratory flow (MEF) in asthmatic patients. It is also effective in decreasing uterine activity during the second and third trimesters. In pregnant ewes and baboons uterine blood flow is not decreased by the doses required to inhibit premature labor.

Terbutaline has a variety of other effects. It increases heart rate, stroke volume, and pulse pressure. It also may cause hyperglycemia and an increase in free fatty acids and glycerol. It may reduce gastrointestinal tone and motility and cause mild general central nervous system stimulation.

ABSORPTION AND BIOTRANSFORMATION

Approximately 30%–55% of an oral dose is absorbed from the gastrointestinal tract. Terbutaline is metabolized in the liver, primarily to an inactive sulfated conjugate, and after being metabolized is excreted in the urine. Only 1% of a subcutaneously administered dose is recovered from bile, indicating the absence of a significant enterohepatic circulation. Excretion of the drug and its metabolites is essentially complete within 72–96 hours after the administration of a single parenteral or oral dose.

RECOMMENDED READING

Andersson, K. E., Bengtsson, L. P., Gustafson, I., and Ingemarsson, I. The relaxing effect of terbutaline on the human uterus during term labor. *Am. J. Obstet. Gynecol.* 121:602–609, 1975.

Andersson, K. E., Bengtsson, L. P., and Ingemarsson, I. Terbutaline inhibition of midtrimester uterine activity induced by prostaglandin $F_{2\alpha}$ and hypertonic saline. *Br. J. Obstet. Gynaecol.* 82:745–749, 1975.

Arner, B. A comparative clinical trial of different subcutaneous doses of terbutaline and orciprenaline in bronchial asthma. *Acta Med. Scand.* 512(Suppl):45–48, 1970.

Arner, B., Bertler, A., Karlefors, T., and Westling, H. Circulatory effects of orciprenaline, adrenaline and a new sympathomimetic β-receptor-stimulating agent, terbutaline, in normal human subjects. *Acta Med. Scand.* 512(Suppl):25–32, 1970.

Carlstrom, S., and Westling, H. Metabolic, circulatory and respiratory effects of a new sympathomimetic β-receptor-stimulating agent, terbutaline, compared with those of orciprenaline. *Acta Med. Scand.* 512(Suppl):33–40, 1970.

Hodach, R. J., Hodach, A. E., Fallon, J. F., Folts, J. D., Bruyere, H. J., and Gilbert, E. F.   The role of β-adrenergic activity in the production of cardiac and aortic arch anomalies in chick embryos. *Teratology* 12:33–46, 1975.

Ingemarsson, I.   Effect of terbutaline on premature labor. A double-blind placebo-controlled study. *Am. J. Obstet. Gynecol.* 125:520–524, 1976.

Sackner, M. A., Dougherty, R., Watson, H., and Wanner, A.   Hemodynamic effects of epinephrine and terbutaline in normal man. *Chest* 68:616–624, 1975.

(RJR)

Tetracylines: Demeclocycline (Declomycin®), Oxytetracycline (Terramycin®), Tetracycline (Achromycin®, Sumycin®)

INDICATIONS AND RECOMMENDATIONS

Tetracyclines are contraindicated during pregnancy. These broad-spectrum antibiotics cross the placenta and are deposited in fetal teeth and bones. Because of adverse effects on these fetal organs, and potential maternal hepatotoxicity, other antibiotics should be used in the pregnant woman.

The deciduous teeth begin to mineralize at approximately 14 weeks of gestation. This process continues until 2 to 3 months after birth. Staining of deciduous teeth is most likely when tetracyclines are administered after the twenty-fifth week.

In one study, when tetracycline was administered to premature newborns a 40% depression of normal skeletal growth resulted. Although this process was rapidly reversed by discontinuing the drug, chronic tetracycline use by a pregnant woman in the third trimester can be expected to have an effect upon fetal bone growth.

Hepatotoxicity (acute fatty liver and, in some cases, death) has been reported in pregnant women treated with tetracyclines in large doses (usually administered intravenously for pyelonephritis).

Occasionally tetracyclines are inadvertently taken during the first trimester. Although these drugs have been associated with congenital anomalies in rats, the data pertaining to humans are, at best, anecdotal. While tetracycline is not recommended for the pregnant woman, the data currently available do not support a recommendation for abortion if inadvertent first trimester exposure occurs.

RECOMMENDED READING

Carter, M. P., and Wilson, F. Antibiotics and congenital malformations. *Lancet* 1:2367–2378, 1963.

Cohlan, S. Q., Bevelander, G., and Tiamsie, T. Growth inhibition of prematures receiving tetracycline. *Am. J. Dis. Child.* 103:453–461, 1963.

Goodman, L. S., and Gilman, A. *The Pharmacological Basis of Therapeutics* (5th ed.). New York: Macmillan, 1975. Pp. 1194–1200.

Harley, J. D., Farrar, J. F., Gray, J. B., and Dunlop, I. C. Aromatic drugs and congenital cataracts. *Lancet* 1:472–473, 1964.

Kucers, A., and Bennett, N. McK. *The Use of Antibiotics* (2nd ed.). London: William Heinemann, 1975. Pp. 381–416.

Kunelis, C. T., Peters, J. L., and Edmondson, H. A. Fatty liver of pregnancy and its relationship to tetracycline therapy. *Am. J. Med.* 38:359–377, 1967.

Whalley, P. J., Adams, R. H., and Combes, B. Tetracycline toxicity in pregnancy. *J.A.M.A.* 189:357–362, 1964.

(DRC)

Theophylline and Aminophylline (Aminodur®, Elixophyllin®, Slo-Phyllin®, Somophyllin®, Theo-Dur®)

INDICATIONS AND RECOMMENDATIONS

Theophylline is safe to use during pregnancy. It is a bronchodilator and the drug of choice for the treatment of asthma in pregnant patients. Theophylline may also be used as an adjunctive agent in the therapy of acute pulmonary edema and in some cases of Cheyne-Stokes respirations.

Blood levels should be monitored in patients receiving theophylline by any route, but clinical response should be the main guide to therapy. When the drug is administered orally, peak and trough levels should be monitored. Patients given the drug intravenously should undergo cardiac monitoring. Appropriate adjustment of dosage should be made in patients with congestive heart failure and severe liver impairment.

Neonates exposed to theophylline in utero as well as those ingesting it in breast milk should be observed for evidence of toxicity. Breastfeeding women should nurse their infants just prior to taking the drug in order to decrease the quantity of drug passing over to the neonate.

SPECIAL CONSIDERATIONS IN PREGNANCY

There are no pharmacokinetic studies of the use of theophylline during pregnancy. The therapeutic goal when this drug is administered is to reverse bronchoconstriction with the lowest dose of theophylline possible. The binding affinity of plasma protein in pregnant women and newborn infants for many drugs is decreased. Since unbound drugs in plasma are generally considered to be the pharmacologically active fractions, a more intense response may be obtained in pregnant women than in their nonpregnant counterparts at similar plasma theophylline concentrations.

Theophylline appears to be mutagenic only in lower organisms. This may be due to the inability of those animals to demethylate this compound, a process that takes place readily in humans. A single case report has described chromosomal abnormalities in association with ingestion of theophylline by the mother, but this remains an isolated occurrence to date. Examination of the limited available data appears to support the impression that teratogenesis with theophylline is negligible.

Toxicity can occur in breastfed infants or by transplacental passage of the drug. Toxic levels have not been well defined and vary from infant to infant. Symptoms may include vomiting, feeding difficulties, jitteriness, tachycardia, cardiac arrhythmias, and transient hyperglycemia. Theophylline concentration in breast milk reaches its peak 1–3 hours after an oral dose. The milk concentration parallels the serum concentration at a mean milk-serum ratio of 0.73. The drug is not bound to protein in breast milk.

DOSAGE

The therapeutic range for theophylline in plasma is 10–20 μg/ml in the nonpregnant woman. Lower levels may possibly suffice during pregnancy. Doses should be adjusted downward for patients with liver disease or congestive heart failure.

The only intravenous preparation available is aminophylline (theophylline ethylenediamine), which is 86% theophylline by weight. It has been recommended that in the treatment of status asthmaticus a loading dose of 6 mg/kg given over 20 minutes be followed by a maintenance infusion of 0.9 mg/kg/hour. If the patient continues to have bronchospasm and does not have signs of toxicity, a further increase can be attempted if plasma levels are not in the therapeutic range. After a bolus dose of 3 mg/kg given over 20 minutes, the maintenance infusion rate may be increased to 1.3–1.5 mg/kg/hour depending on the plasma level. If the patient has been taking theophylline orally in adequate amounts, half the loading dose described above and the same maintenance dosage should be administered. If she has been taking the drug erratically, it is probably best to proceed as if she were not taking it at all.

Oral theophylline is used for the long-term treatment of bronchospasm. Plain, enteric-coated, and sustained-release preparations are available. The use of enteric-coated preparations is not recommended as absorption is unpredictable. Plain theophylline or aminophylline tablets or liquids are usually taken every 6 hours. Sustained-release preparations have the advantage of an 8–12-hour dose interval.

Theophylline can be given rectally as either a suppository or a solution. The use of suppositories is not recommended as they tend to be absorbed erratically and can produce unpredictable and dangerous blood levels. Rectal solutions are more predictably absorbed and produce less proctitis. Rectal solutions may be administered as follows: aminophylline solution 300 mg/5 ml every 8–12 hours, or theophylline monoethanolamine 250 mg/30 ml or 500 mg/30 ml every 8–12 hours.

ADVERSE EFFECTS

Side effects and toxicity are related in most cases to plasma concentrations of the drug. They are usually of minor significance when the drug is maintained within the usual therapeutic range. Side effects include anorexia, nausea, vomiting, diuresis, and abdominal distention. Palpitations and sinus and atrial tachycardias may occur. Precordial pain and hypotension have been reported with rapid intravenous administration of aminophylline. Excitation, anxiety, insomnia, diaphoresis, tremor, and even convulsions may occur. The latter is a toxic phenomenon and is usually seen with plasma levels close to 60 μg/ml.

MECHANISM OF ACTION

The actions of theophylline are mediated through its inhibition of phosphodiesterase, the enzyme responsible for the degradation of cyclic adenosine monophosphate (AMP). Increase in the intracellular concentration of cyclic AMP produces smooth muscle relaxation.

The primary action of theophylline is to relax bronchiolar smooth muscle, especially when it is in spasm. It also sensitizes the respiratory center to carbon dioxide, causing an increase in both respiratory rate and depth. It has both inotropic and chronotropic effects on the myocardium and causes vasodilation in the pulmonary, coronary, and systemic circulations. Cardiac output is increased and venous filling pressure is reduced. Theophylline is a central nervous system stimulant and has been used to treat apnea in the premature infant. It also increases gastric secretion and decreases small and large bowel motility. In addition, catecholamine release may be stimulated.

ABSORPTION AND BIOTRANSFORMATION

Ninety percent of an oral dose reaches the circulation, and absorption is better in the fasting state. Peak concentrations are achieved between 1 and 3 hours after administration of uncoated tablets and in 30 minutes with elixir and solutions. Theophylline is metabolized by the liver and excreted in the urine. Sixty percent of the drug is bound to plasma proteins at therapeutic concentrations. It does not displace bilirubin from albumin. The half-life is usually 4–5 hours in adults but may be elevated in patients with liver disease or congestive failure.

RECOMMENDED READING

Mitenko, P. A., and Ogilvie, R. I. Pharmacokinetics of intravenous theophylline. *Clin. Pharmacol. Ther.* 14:509–513, 1973.

Mitenko, P. A., and Ogilvie, R. I. Rational intravenous doses of theophylline. *N. Engl. J. Med.* 289:600–603, 1973.

Mitenko, P. A., and Ogilvie, R. I. Bioavailability and efficacy of a sustained release theophylline tablet. *Clin. Pharmacol. Ther.* 16:720–726, 1974.

Salem, H., and Jackson, R. H. Oral theophylline preparations—a review of their clinical efficacy in the treatment of bronchial asthma. *Ann. Allergy* 32:189–199, 1974.

Timson, J. Theobromine-theophylline. *Mutat. Res.* 32:169–178, 1975.

Yeh, T. F., and Pildes, R. S. Transplacental aminophylline toxicity in a neonate (Letter). *Lancet* 1:910, 1977.

Yurchak, A. M., and Jusko, W. J. Theophylline secretion into breast milk. *Pediatrics* 57:518–520, 1976.

(RJR)

Tobacco

INDICATIONS AND RECOMMENDATIONS

The use of tobacco is contraindicated during pregnancy. This drug is the dried leaf of the *Nicotiana tabacum* plant, and a widely used agent that is smoked by approximately one-third of American women of childbearing age. An estimated 20%–25% of women smoke throughout pregnancy. Tobacco has no known therapeutic uses.

Cigarette smoking should be actively discouraged in anyone but especially in pregnant women. Even if a habituated person cannot stop smoking completely, there is good evidence to show that she should try to decrease her cigarette consumption to less than seven per day.

Lactating women also should be discouraged from smoking and should smoke as little as possible if they cannot achieve complete abstinence.

SPECIAL CONSIDERATIONS IN PREGNANCY

A growing body of data links cigarette smoking to complications of pregnancy. Every investigator who has looked at the relationship of birth weight to cigarette smoking has confirmed that offspring of smoking mothers have lower birth weights than those of nonsmokers. Although the actual difference in birth weight is only in the range of a few hundred grams, every study shows a statistically significant difference in these weights. Studies that correct for gestational age confirm this finding. Not only have smokers been shown to have smaller offspring than nonsmokers, but over thirty investigations have indicated that they also have twice the number of growth-retarded babies.

This effect of smoking seems to be dose-related as well as related to the stage of pregnancy in which smoking occurs. If a woman stops smoking prior to the end of the fourth month of pregnancy, it is probable that her offspring will not differ significantly in weight from that of a nonsmoker. Furthermore, women who smoke less than seven to ten cigarettes per day tend to have children whose birth weights do not differ significantly from those of nonsmokers. The direct causative factor in cigarette smoke that leads to decreased birth weight is not clear, although animal studies show that prolonged exposure to elevated levels of carbon monoxide will cause lowering of birth weight.

Both retrospective and prospective studies strongly suggest that cigarette smoking is related to an increased incidence of spontaneous abortion, although most of these studies do not adequately control for confounding variables. A report by Kline and associates, however, attempted to control for many of these variables and revealed a nearly twofold greater risk of spontaneous abortion in smokers over nonsmokers.

Cigarette smoking is most obviously related to stillbirth in women with other complicating problems, including low socio-economic status and poor previous obstetric history. In the United States, for example, black women have more stillbirths than white women, and cigarette smoking magnifies this difference. Animal studies have shown that nicotine and some other cigarette components may significantly increase the incidence of stillbirths.

In large studies from both England and Canada the perinatal mortality for infants of smokers was significantly higher than that for infants of nonsmokers. The Canadian study showed a highly significant dose-response relationship. In addition, the British study demonstrated a significant relationship between smoking after the fourth month of pregnancy and increased perinatal mortality. Patients who gave up smoking by the fourth month were found to reduce the risk of perinatal mortality to that of nonsmokers. In addition, this study showed that smoking in patients of low socioeconomic strata caused an even higher than expected increase in perinatal mortality. The same association has been made with regard to poor obstetric history combined with smoking.

The perinatal mortality for infants under 2,500 gm born to smokers is less than that of nonsmokers. The reason seems to be that these infants are primarily small for gestational age rather than premature. However, for infants of comparable gestational age, the mortality is higher for the offspring of smokers than nonsmokers.

Several epidemiological studies reveal a significant decrease in the incidence of preeclampsia in smokers. This appears to be inversely proportional to the amount the woman smokes. However, there is data to show that if a smoker does develop preeclampsia, her infant is at higher risk than that of a nonsmoker.

In one study of 2,000 women there was a definite trend (though not statistically significant) toward inadequate breast milk production in smoking mothers as compared to nonsmoking controls. It has been shown that nicotine is excreted in milk in amounts proportional to the quantity consumed by the mother. Several cases of nicotine poisoning in nursing infants of mothers smoking twenty to forty cigarettes per day have been reported.

ADVERSE EFFECTS

Among the many medical conditions clearly associated with ingestion of cigarette smoke are: mucosal epitheliomas; lung cancer; cancers of the oropharyngeal cavity, esophagus, and larynx; emphysema; "smokers respiratory syndrome"; coronary artery disease; cerebrovascular disease; cardiac arrhythmias; and peripheral vascular disease.

Nicotine has parasympathetic effects on the gastrointestinal tract, occasionally resulting in diarrhea and often leading to decreased intestinal motility. It can cause respiratory depression and arrest by its action of blocking the neuromuscular junction of respiratory muscles. Furthermore, a minor central nervous system (CNS) paralysis may occur. Other CNS effects such as tremors (at low doses) and convulsions (at higher doses) can be reversed with antiparkinsonism drugs, curariform drugs, adrenergic blockers, hypnotics, and anticonvulsants. Nicotine also has an antidiuretic effect mediated through release of antidiuretic hormone (ADH).

MECHANISM OF ACTION

Nearly 500 compounds have been isolated from tobacco smoke. These include several chemicals irritating to mucous membranes; polonium-210 and nickel, which have been implicated in lung cancer; and carbon monoxide, which makes up approximately 1% of cigarette smoke by volume. The major active component of tobacco, however, is nicotine, which comprises an average of 6–8 mg per cigarette. Approximately 90% of the nicotine in inhaled tobacco smoke is systemically absorbed.

Nicotine, a toxic substance that acts on a variety of neuroeffector junctions, has both stimulant and depressant phases of action. Its net effect therefore is the algebraic summation of those actions. These are usually dose-related and depend on time since ingestion. An initial stimulatory effect is usually followed by a depressant effect. This pattern occurs in all autonomic ganglia and is responsible for many if not most of the effects of nicotine.

In general, nicotine will increase heart rate and blood pressure and its cardiovascular effects parallel those of sympathetic stimulation. The sympathomimetic effects can be negated by catecholamine blockers, which implies that they are mediated through the adrenal glands and other catecholamine-releasing organs.

ABSORPTION AND BIOTRANSFORMATION

Nicotine, the major component of tobacco smoke, is absorbed from oral and gastrointestinal mucosa, the respiratory tract, and skin. Eighty to ninety percent is detoxified by the liver, kidney, and lungs; then the remainder plus the detoxification products are excreted through the kidney. This occurs most expeditiously in acidified urine. Nicotine is also excreted in the milk of lactating women in direct proportion to the amount of tobacco consumed. The milk may contain as much as 0.5 mg/liter.

RECOMMENDED READING

Goodman, L. S., and Gilman, A. *The Pharmacological Basis of Therapeutics* (5th ed.). New York: Macmillan, 1975. Pp. 588–592.

Kline, J., Stein, Z. A., and Susser, M. Smoking: A risk factor for spontaneous abortion. *N. Engl. J. Med.* 297:793–796, 1977.

U.S. Public Health Service. *The Health Consequences of Smoking. A Report of the Surgeon General.* Washington, D.C.: U.S. Government Printing Office, 1973.

(AJF)

Tolazoline (Priscoline®)

INDICATIONS AND RECOMMENDATIONS

Tolazoline is relatively contraindicated during pregnancy because other therapeutic agents are preferable. Tolazoline, like phentolamine, is an alpha-adrenergic blocker. In addition to its alpha blocking effects, it has a variety of nonrelated sympathomimetic, parasympathomimetic, and histaminic actions. There are no clear-cut indications for its use during pregnancy.

Tolazoline produces vasodilation and cardiac stimulation, which usually results in a rise in systemic blood pressure. It can produce tachycardias and arrhythmias. Although the drug has been used to treat neonates for pulmonary hypertension, little is known of its effects when administered during pregnancy. In one study, neonates given tolazoline showed complications of gastrointestinal hemorrhage, thrombocytopenia, and transient renal failure.

There are few documented indications for the use of tolazoline. The most favorable clinical responses have been described with early Raynaud's syndrome. However, because tolazoline has had limited use in pregnancy, it cannot be recommended.

RECOMMENDED READING

Goetzman, B. W., Sunshine, P., Johnson, J. D., Wennberg, R. P., Hackel, A., Merten, D. F., Bartoletti, A. L., and Silverman, N. H. Neonatal hypoxia and pulmonary vasospasm response to tolazoline. *J. Pediatr.* 89:617–621, 1976.

Goodman, L. S., and Gilman, A. *The Pharmacological Basis of Therapeutics* (5th ed.). New York: Macmillan, 1975. Pp. 541–543.

(MJM)

Triamterene (Dyrenium®)

INDICATIONS AND RECOMMENDATIONS

Triamterene is relatively contraindicated during pregnancy because other therapeutic agents are preferable. It is a potassium-sparing diuretic that acts directly on tubular transport in the distal tubule. It is not an aldosterone antagonist.

The effects of the drug on uterine blood flow and the fetus have not been well studied.

If diuretics are necessary during pregnancy, the thiazides or furosemide are preferable to triamterene. Serum potassium levels should be followed closely whenever pregnant women are given diuretics. If hypokalemia develops, oral potassium supplementation will effectively correct this problem. This drug, therefore, has no important advantage over others whose effects in pregnancy are better known.

RECOMMENDED READING

Gifford, R. W., Jr. A guide to the practical use of diuretics. *J.A.M.A.* 235:1890–1893, 1976.

Goodman, L. S., and Gilman, A. *The Pharmacological Basis of Therapeutics* (5th ed.). New York: Macmillan, 1975. Pp. 838–839.

(PCL)

Tricyclic Antidepressants: Amitriptyline (Elavil®), Desipramine (Norpramin®), Doxepin (Sinequan®), Imipramine (Tofranil®), Nortriptyline (Aventyl®, Pamelor®), Protriptyline (Vivactil®)

INDICATIONS AND RECOMMENDATIONS

The use of tricyclic antidepressants during pregnancy should be limited to the treatment of those women who clearly require the medication for psychiatric indications, especially endogenous depression of abrupt onset. Reactive depression and depression accompanied by anxiety are less likely to be relieved by these drugs and therefore do not indicate their use during pregnancy. It does not appear that any member of this family of drugs is the agent of choice for use during pregnancy.

SPECIAL CONSIDERATIONS IN PREGNANCY

Animal studies have shown that the tricyclic antidepressants cross the placenta slowly.

There have been isolated cases of infants born to women who received tricyclic antidepressants immediately prior to delivery who have reportedly suffered from heart failure, tachycardia, myoclonus, respiratory distress, and urinary retention. Withdrawal symptoms have been observed in infants whose mothers were treated with imipramine during the antenatal period. Use of the tricyclic antidepressants has been associated with congenital malformations, although a causal relationship has not been proved.

The excretion of these drugs in breast milk is not significant.

DOSAGE

Doses of the tricyclic antidepressants must be individualized. After an initial dose has been given, dosage is gradually increased over 1 to 2 weeks to the maintenance dose that will provide maximal efficacy and minimal side effects. Table 13 details recommended dosages of these antidepressants.

ADVERSE EFFECTS

Sedation is the most prominent initial effect of the tricyclic antidepressants, the magnitude of which depends on the individual agent. Other side effects include tachycardia and orthostatic hypotension. These agents have potent anticholinergic activity

Table 13. Recommended Dosages of the Tricyclic Antidepressants

Drug	Usual Daily Starting Dose (mg)	Usual Daily Maintenance Dosage Range (mg)
Amitriptyline	50–75	75–300
Desipramine	50–75	75–300
Doxepin	50–75	75–300
Imipramine	50–75	75–300
Nortriptyline	75	40–100
Protriptyline	10	10–40

and commonly cause dry mouth, blurred vision, urinary retention, and constipation. Allergic reactions, inappropriate secretion of antidiuretic hormone, and galactorrhea are only encountered rarely. Toxicity due to acute overdosage is characterized by hyperpyrexia, hypertension, seizures, and coma.

MECHANISM OF ACTION

The tricyclic antidepressants block the reuptake of neurotransmitters, including norepinephrine and seratonin, in adrenergic nerve endings. The resulting increased concentration of neurotransmitter at the receptor is postulated to be responsible for the therapeutic effects of these agents.

ABSORPTION AND BIOTRANSFORMATION

The tricyclic antidepressants are well absorbed from the gastrointestinal tract; they are metabolized in the liver. They and their metabolites are excreted in urine and feces.

RECOMMENDED READING

American Hospital Formulary Service. *Monographs for Amitriptyline HCl* (1967), *Desipramine HCl* (1965), *Doxepin HCl* (1970), *Imipramine HCl* (1962). Washington, D.C.: American Society of Hospital Pharmacists, 1962, 1965, 1967, 1970.

Goodman, L. S., and Gilman, A. *The Pharmacological Basis of Therapeutics* (5th ed.). New York: Macmillan, 1975. Pp. 174–179.

Hollister, L. E. Doxepin hydrochloride. *Ann. Int. Med.* 81:360–363, 1974.

The Neuropharmacology of Depression. Merrell-National Laboratories, Cincinnati, Ohio, July, 1977.

(JMH)

Trimethadione (Tridione®)

INDICATIONS AND RECOMMENDATIONS

Trimethadione is relatively contraindicated during pregnancy because other therapeutic agents are preferable. It is a second-line anticonvulsant used in the treatment of petit mal epilepsy. It has been associated with teratogenic effects in the human fetus. A report of 4 women who used trimethadione during the first trimester of 14 pregnancies revealed 8 children with developmental defects (4 facial cleft defects and 4 cardiac defects), 3 spontaneous abortions, and 3 normal children. In addition, a fetal trimethadione syndrome has been described, consisting of mild mental retardation, V-shaped eyebrows, speech difficulties, palatal anomalies, abnormal ears, and epicanthus. If treatment for petit mal epilepsy is required during pregnancy, ethosuximide is preferred.

RECOMMENDED READING

Eadie, M. J., and Tyrer, J. H. *Anticonvulsant Therapy.* Edinburgh: Churchill-Livingstone, 1974.

German, J., Kowal, A., and Ehlers, K. H. Trimethadione and human teratogenesis. *Teratology* 3:349–361, 1970.

Goodman, L. S., and Gilman, A. *The Pharmacological Basis of Therapeutics* (5th ed.). New York: Macmillan, 1975. Pp. 214–216.

Tuchmann-Duplessis, H. *Drug Effects on the Fetus.* Sydney, Australia: Adis Press, 1975.

Woodbury, D. M., Penry, J. K., and Schmidt, R. P. *Antiepileptic Drugs.* New York: Raven Press, 1972.

Zackai, E. H., Mellman, W. J., Neiderer, B., and Hanson, J. W. The fetal trimethadione syndrome. *J. Pediatr.* 87:280–284, 1975.

(PHR)

Trimethaphan (Arfonad®)

INDICATIONS AND RECOMMENDATIONS

The use of trimethaphan is relatively contraindicated during pregnancy because other therapeutic agents are preferable. It is a ganglionic blocker that acts almost immediately as an antihypertensive agent. Its therapeutic action is so evanescent that it must be given by continuous infusion.

Trimethaphan prevents the attachment of acetylcholine released by the preganglionic neuron to the receptor sites of the postganglionic axon. This results in the inhibition of both sympathetic and parasympathetic impulses.

Decreased intravascular volume or any drug that inhibits sympathetic activity will augment the antihypertensive action of this drug. Furthermore, the hypotensive action of trimethaphan is accompanied by a decrease in glomerular filtration rate.

Side effects include the many problems that accompany ganglionic blockade, most importantly obstipation and urinary retention. In addition, administration of ganglionic blockers to the mother has been associated with meconium ileus in the neonate.

Trimethaphan should not be used during pregnancy unless other more acceptable agents have proved unsuccessful.

RECOMMENDED READING

Koch-Weser, J. Hypertensive emergencies. *N. Engl. J. Med.* 290:211–214, 1974.

Martin, J. D. A critical survey of drugs used in the treatment of hypertensive crises of pregnancy. *Med. J. Aust.* 2:252–254, 1974.

The treatment of malignant hypertension and hypertensive emergencies. A statement by the AMA Committee on Hypertension. *J.A.M.A.* 228:1673–1679, 1974.

(RLB)

Trimethobenzamide (Tigan®)

INDICATIONS AND RECOMMENDATIONS

Trimethobenzamide is safe to use during pregnancy. The usual therapeutic dosages may be used for treatment of nausea and vomiting during pregnancy.

SPECIAL CONSIDERATIONS IN PREGNANCY

Large-scale prospective studies assessing the use of trimethobenzamide in pregnancy have failed to show an increased risk of malformation in the fetus at normal doses.

DOSAGE

The usual adult oral dose of trimethobenzamide is 250 mg two to three times a day. The IM and rectal dose is 200 mg three to four times a day.

ADVERSE EFFECTS

At recommended dosages, side effects are relatively uncommon; they include drowsiness and dizziness, and local irritation if the IM or rectal route is used.

MECHANISM OF ACTION

The exact mechanism of action of trimethobenzamide as an antiemetic is obscure. It is thought to depress the chemoreceptor trigger zone. It does not suppress the vomiting center or block visceral impulses to the vomiting center. It is structurally related to the antihistamines but has only weak antihistaminic activity.

ABSORPTION AND BIOTRANSFORMATION

Trimethobenzamide is well absorbed after oral administration. Measurable blood levels may persist for as long as 24 hours.

Within 72 hours, 30%–50% of the administered dose is excreted unchanged in the urine. Trimethobenzamide may also be metabolized in the liver and its metabolites excreted in bile and urine.

RECOMMENDED READING

Heinonen, D., Slone, D., and Shapiro, S. (Eds.). *Birth Defects and Drugs in Pregnancy.* Littleton, Mass.: Publishing Sciences Group, 1977. Pp. 323–330.

Long, J. W. *Essential Guide to Prescription Drugs.* New York: Harper & Row, 1977. Pp. 641–643.

Milkovich, L., and vanDenBerg, B. J. An evaluation of the teratogenicity of certain antinauseant drugs. *Am. J. Obstet. Gynecol.* 125:244–248, 1976.

Pearlman, D. S. Antihistamines: Pharmacology and clinical use. *Drugs* 12:258–273, 1976.

(DJK)

Tripelennamine (Pyribenzamine®, PBZ®)

INDICATIONS AND RECOMMENDATIONS

The use of tripelennamine during pregnancy should be limited to the treatment of allergic symptoms caused by histamine release, including urticaria, rhinitis, and pruritus. Whenever possible, however, the primary treatment for such symptoms should be avoidance of the allergen. This drug should be avoided by breastfeeding women.

SPECIAL CONSIDERATIONS IN PREGNANCY

No prospective studies that evaluate the safety of tripelennamine's use during pregnancy have been conducted. One large retrospective study, however, found no evidence incriminating tripelennamine as a teratogenic agent.

Because of its anticholinergic properties, tripelennamine may inhibit lactation. In addition, small amounts may be secreted into breast milk. This and all antihistamines should therefore be avoided by the lactating mother.

DOSAGE

The adult dose of tripelennamine hydrochloride is 50–100 mg every 4–6 hours. An extended-release preparation is available and may be prescribed in a dose of 100 mg every 8–12 hours. Tripelennamine citrate is available in an elixir; 37.5 mg of the citrate is equivalent to 25 mg of the hydrochloride.

ADVERSE EFFECTS

Anticholinergic side effects are the most common. These include dry mouth and eyes, and, rarely, blurred vision. Drowsiness, anorexia, nausea, epigastric distress, and dizziness also may be seen.

MECHANISM OF ACTION

Tripelennamine is a competitive antagonist of histamine that decreases edema formation by diminishing capillary dilatation and permeability. It merely provides palliative, not curative, therapy for allergic symptoms. It has anticholinergic activity, produces drowsiness, and possesses local anesthetic activity when applied topically.

ABSORPTION AND BIOTRANSFORMATION

The drug is primarily metabolized in the liver, probably by hydroxylation followed by glucuronidation. Excretion is via the kidney.

RECOMMENDED READING

Goodman, L. S., and Gilman, A. *The Pharmacological Basis of Therapeutics* (5th ed.). New York: Macmillan, 1975. P. 609.

Greenberger, P., and Patterson, R. Safety of therapy for allergic symptoms during pregnancy. *Ann. Intern. Med.* 89:234–237, 1978.

Heinonen, O. P., Slone, D., and Shapiro, S. *Birth Defects and Drugs in Pregnancy.* Littleton, Mass.: Publishing Sciences Group, 1977. Pp. 323–324.

Nishimura, H., and Tanimura, T. *Aspects of the Teratogenicity of Drugs.* Amsterdam: Excerpta Medica, 1976.

(JRC)

Vancomycin (Vancocin®)

INDICATIONS AND RECOMMENDATIONS

The use of vancomycin during pregnancy should be limited to the treatment of life-threatening infections in patients allergic to penicillin, or to treatment of serious staphylococcal infections caused by strains resistant to penicillinase-resistant penicillins or cephalosporins.

SPECIAL CONSIDERATIONS IN PREGNANCY

Because of potential ototoxicity to the fetus, vancomycin should be used only when specifically indicated.

DOSAGE

The usual dose is 2 gm/day intravenously, being divided into doses given every 6 hours or every 12 hours. If creatinine clearance is 50–80 ml/min, the dose should be given every 1–3 days. If the creatinine clearance is 10–50 ml/min, the dose is given every 3–10 days. If the creatinine clearance is less than 10 ml/min, only 1 gm is given every 7 days.

ADVERSE EFFECTS

Frequent side effects include thrombophlebitis, chills, and fever. Vancomycin can also be nephrotoxic and ototoxic, particularly with large doses or prolonged use (more than 10 days). It may also have these effects in the presence of renal impairment or in the elderly. Rare reactions include peripheral neuropathy and urticaria.

MECHANISM OF ACTION

Vancomycin is a bacteriocidal antibiotic that acts by inhibiting cell wall synthesis. It is active against streptococci, staphylococci, enterococci, *Corynebacteria,* and *Clostridia.*

ABSORPTION AND BIOTRANSFORMATION

Vancomycin is poorly absorbed orally, with large quantities excreted in the stool. It is used intravenously, with 80% of an injected dose excreted by the kidney. In the presence of renal insufficiency dangerously high blood concentrations may occur.

RECOMMENDED READING

Davis, D. M. *Textbook of Adverse Drug Reactions.* Oxford: Oxford University Press, 1977. P. 70.
Handbook of Antimicrobial Therapy. The Medical Letter on Drugs and Therapeutics (Rev. ed.). New Rochelle, N.Y.: The Medical Letter, 1978.

(GRD)

Xanthines (over-the-counter): Caffeine, Theobromine, Theophylline

INDICATIONS AND RECOMMENDATIONS

Xanthines in the quantities present in coffee, tea, cocoa, and cola-flavored drinks are probably safe during pregnancy, if consumed in moderation, in the absence of peptic ulcer or hypertensive heart disease. A recent FDA study has linked large doses of caffeine (human equivalent of 20–24 cups of coffee daily), administered as a bolus via nasogastric tube to pregnant rats, with missing digits in the offspring. There is no known teratogenicity when beverages containing xanthines are drunk during human pregnancy.

In a review by Anderson it is stated that 6 hours after a mother consumes caffeine the level in breast milk is only 1% of the total dose. Breastfed infants whose mothers are ingesting xanthines, however, may become irritable, sleep poorly, or develop gastrointestinal colic. It is recommended therefore that nursing mothers limit their intake of coffee or tea to 2 cups per day or less.

SPECIAL CONSIDERATIONS IN PREGNANCY

The xanthines produce no unique effects in the mother during pregnancy. The fetus may be subject to stimulation of its central nervous system (CNS) or skeletal musculature, or both, which results in an increase in activity in utero. Fetal cardiac stimulation may cause tachycardia or premature contractions. Xanthines have caused chromosomal breakage in some microorganisms and in fruit flies. Breakage in human chromosome preparations, however, has only been observed with doses far greater than those obtainable from drinking coffee or tea. Similarly, teratogenicity in rats has been demonstrated only with large bolus doses administered by nasogastric tube. Until more data are available, it is probably best for pregnant women to limit their caffeine intake, although no threshold dosage has been defined.

Caffeine reaches detectable levels in the blood of nursing infants. Jitteriness has been reported in an infant whose mother had a history of heavy caffeine use. Children and infants are more sensitive to the effects of xanthines than adults.

DOSAGE

1. Coffee and tea contain 100–150 mg of caffeine per average cup.
2. Nondietetic cola drinks contain 35–55 mg of caffeine per 12-ounce glass.
3. Dietetic drinks in some cases contain unstated amounts of caffeine.
4. Cocoa contains approximately 200 mg of theobromine per cup.
5. Tea contains theophylline in varying amounts.

ADVERSE EFFECTS

The fatal dose of caffeine is 10 grams. It is quite unlikely that this amount will be ingested, however, because reactions usually begin after 1 gram has been consumed. CNS side effects include restlessness and disturbed sleep patterns, tremor, tinnitus, and excitement, which may progress to delirium. Tachycardia and arrhythmias may occur. Other side effects include diuresis, dyspepsia, and nausea and vomiting. Theophylline may be fatal to adults, but only if administered intravenously. Children, however, have been fatally intoxicated by pharmacological preparations of theophylline administered orally, rectally, or parenterally. In adults theophylline may cause headaches, palpitations, nausea, and hypotension.

MECHANISM OF ACTION

The xanthines affect many systems in the body by increasing intracellular cyclic adenosine monophosphate, altering ionic calcium levels, and potentiating the action of catecholamines. CNS, respiratory, and skeletal muscle effects are greatest for caffeine, less for theophylline, and least for theobromine. Smooth muscle relaxation, coronary artery dilation, myocardial stimulation, and diuresis, on the other hand, are related to theophylline, theobromine, and caffeine, in decreasing order of potency. Excitation of the CNS on all levels results from ingestion of 150–250 mg of caffeine (1–2 cups of coffee). This is manifested by reduced drowsiness, increased motor activity, a reflex excitability, and awareness of sensory stimuli, as well as stimulation of respiratory, vasomotor, and vagal centers. Theophylline increases reflex excitability and the rate and depth of respirations.

The xanthines directly stimulate the myocardium and increase cardiac output. Heart rate may be slowed secondary to medullary vagal center stimulation but is increased with large doses. Blood vessels are usually dilated by these agents, but there may be an increase in cerebral vascular resistance. Although bronchial and bile duct musculature are relaxed, there is an increase in the strength of skeletal muscle contraction. Glomerular filtration rate and renal blood flow are increased, with a resultant diuresis and increase in sodium and chloride excretion. Caffeine may increase the amount of gastric acid secretion and aggravate peptic ulcers. The xanthines also cause a slight increase in the basal metabolic rate and in higher concentrations stimulate lipolysis, glyco-genolysis, and gluconeogenesis.

ABSORPTION AND BIOTRANSFORMATION

The xanthines are absorbed after oral, parenteral, or rectal admin-istration. Because caffeine and theophylline have poor aqueous solubility, absorption from the gastrointestinal tract may be erratic, but, when taken orally, their onset of action is usually within 30 minutes. The xanthines are metabolized by partial demethylation and oxidation, but about 10% is excreted unchanged in the urine.

RECOMMENDED READING

Anderson, P. O. Drugs in breast feeding—a review. *Drug Intell. Clin. Pharm.* 11:208–223, 1977.

Goodman, L. S., and Gilman, A. *The Pharmacological Basis of Therapeutics* (5th ed.). New York: Macmillan, 1975. Pp. 367–378.

Nelson, M. M., and Forfar, J. O. Associations between drugs administered during pregnancy and congenital abnormalities of the fetus. *Br. Med. J.* 1:523–527, 1971.

Rivera-Calimlim, L. Drugs in breast milk *Drug Ther.* (Hospital ed.) 8:59–63, 1977.

Schenkel, B., and Vorherr, H. Non-prescription drugs during pregnancy: Potential teratogenic and toxic effects upon embryo and fetus. *J. Reprod. Med.* 12:27–45, 1974.

(RAC)

APPENDIX: VITAMINS AND MINERALS

Vitamins

Water-Soluble Vitamins

FOLIC ACID

Folate and folic acid are nutrients required for pyrimidine metabolism. Folic acid is also used in a number of other reactions in intermediary metabolism, including the conversion of homocysteine to methionine and the metabolism of the histidine nucleus.

Since the blockage of DNA synthesis is the major consequence of folate deficiency, the most rapidly dividing cells are those primarily affected. Bone marrow cells develop megaloblastic changes. The peripheral manifestation of this change is a macrocytic anemia, moderate leukopenia (with hypersegmented neutrophils), and thrombocytopenia.

Folates are present in large quantities in peanuts, liver, kidney, and green leafy vegetables. Cereal and dairy products contain low quantities. These folates are usually supplied as polyglutamates that are cleaved in the intestinal lumen. The monoglutamate form is believed to be absorbed into the bloodstream. Oral contraceptives and phenytoin may affect this metabolism and account, at least in part, for the alterations in folate levels when these medications are used.

Folic acid deficiency is rare except in malabsorption conditions, infancy, and pregnancy. The fetus can apparently extract adequate amounts of folate even in the presence of megaloblastic anemia in the mother. This extraction and possibly the reduced availability of folate produced by intestinal flora accounts for decompensation in pregnant women with a long history of poor dietary intake.

As noted previously, there appears to be an interaction between folic acid and anticonvulsants, most notably phenytoin and phenobarbital. A number of studies have reported an association between low maternal folate levels and congenital malformations. Although prospective studies have failed to confirm this as a causal relationship, it has been implicated as the etiology of teratogenicity in phenytoin-associated malformations. Clinical decision-making is made more difficult by the ability of folic acid supplementation to lower phenytoin blood levels. In some instances a significant rise in the number of seizures has been reported when folate has been given to a patient on phenytoin. In gravid patients on antiepileptic medications, therefore, it is suggested that blood levels of folic acid and anticonvulsants be carefully followed and changes in dosage be made accordingly.

Tissue stores of folate are in the range of 5–10 mg. Nonpregnant women require 50 μg of folate daily, and during pregnancy this rises to 450 μg. A daily dose of 500 μg and 1.0 mg for singleton and twin gestation, respectively, will provide an adequate prophylactic dose of folic acid for mother and fetus during gestation. For treatment of folate deficiency anemia, a daily dose of 1.0 mg with or without a parenteral loading dose is recommended.

THIAMIN (B_1)

Thiamin functions as a coenzyme in carbohydrate metabolism. Dietary deficiency leads to beriberi. Studies have revealed an increased requirement for thiamine during pregnancy if serum levels are to be maintained. One study revealed a 25% incidence of deficiency in biochemical parameters requiring thiamin. The significance of these findings is unclear, however, in that the fetus is able to achieve a higher serum level than the mother.

In view of these studies, the recommended dietary allowance (RDA) of thiamin in pregnancy is 0.1 mg/1000 Kcal greater than the 0.5 mg/1000 Kcal needed by a nonpregnant woman.

RIBOFLAVIN (B_2)

Riboflavin acts as a coenzyme required for the flavoproteins involved in oxidative metabolism. Moderate degrees of deficiency have caused fetal malformations in rodents. No association between deficiency and malformations in humans has been noted.

Recent studies have used levels of erythrocyte glutathione reductase as a measure of riboflavin deficiency. This test measures flavin-adenine-dinucleotide, the major riboflavin coenzyme. These studies have revealed an increasing requirement as pregnancy progresses. This has been clinically confirmed by the manifestations of deficiency (glossitis, angular stomatitis, cheilosis, and corneal vascularization) in the third trimester in mothers with low riboflavin intake.

Despite symptoms in the mother, however, no influence on the outcome of pregnancy could be detected. This maternal/fetal discrepancy may be related to the active transport of riboflavin across the placenta. Cord levels have been reported to be as high as four times those in the mother's serum.

In view of these studies, the RDA includes an intake of 0.3 mg/day during pregnancy above the baseline of 0.6 mg/1000 Kcal/day.

NIACIN

Niacin is the generic name for nicotinic acid and nicotinamide. Nicotinamide functions in coenzymes concerned with glycolysis, fat synthesis, and tissue respiration.

Although pellegra has been found to be associated with dietary deficiency of niacin in areas in which corn is the major source of protein, the relationship between the two is not linear. Some dietary tryptophan can be converted to niacin, and a ratio of 60 mg of tryptophan to 1 mg of niacin has been proposed.

The RDA includes an increase for pregnant women of 2 mg above the basal allowance of 6.6 mg/1000 Kcal. This accounts for the increased allowance of calories during gestation. There have been no controlled studies regarding the influence of dietary deficiency during pregnancy.

PYRIDOXINE (B_6)

Vitamin B_6 is a group of interrelated substances: pyridoxine, pyridoxamine, pyridoxal, and pyridoxal phosphate. Phosphorylated pyridoxal is required as a coenzyme in amino-acid metabolism. A number of conditions have been related to B_6 deficiency; dietary deprivation can result in seizures, hypochromic microcytic anemia, abdominal distress, vomiting, depression, and confusion. The use of certain medications such as penicillamine, isoniazid, and oral contraceptives has been shown to increase the excretion of B_6.

Vitamin B_6 was first administered in 1942 as a treatment for hyperemesis gravidarum. Since that time much controversy has arisen regarding B_6 supplementation during pregnancy. All studies reveal a lower level of B_6-dependent activities during pregnancy. Serum levels fall late in the first trimester and remain depressed throughout pregnancy. A rise to the normal values for nonpregnant women has been noted by the fourth postpartum day.

The placenta actively transports B_6, and studies have revealed high placental levels of pyridoxal kinase. Levels in the fetus are two to three times higher than levels in the mother, but they rise further with increases in the mother's levels. Umbilical vein levels are higher than umbilical artery levels, indicating fetal utilization.

Attempts at normalization of biochemical and excretion indices, as well as serum levels, in pregnant women have suggested that supplementation of 10–15 mg daily is needed. No controlled trials have suggested benefits to the mother or fetus by this type of supplementation.

In view of these difficulties, the RDA includes an increase of 0.5 mg/day above basal requirements of 2.5 mg/day.

CYANOCOBALMIN (B_{12})

Vitamin B_{12} is present in all cells of mammalian tissue. It is essential in nucleic acid metabolism because of its role in allowing 5-methyltetrahydrofolate to return to the utilizable folate pool. Deficiency results in megaloblastosis of the bone marrow and gastrointestinal mucosa as well as in neuronal dysfunction.

The average diet contains 5–15 μg of vitamin B_{12} daily. Absorption via intrinsic factor is quite efficient, and dietary deficiency is very rare, except in strict vegetarians.

Studies have revealed a progressive decline in serum vitamin B_{12} levels during pregnancy. It is unlikely that this represents a true deficiency state but rather is a physiological alteration. The fetus has been shown to concentrate vitamin B_{12}, and cord serum levels are about three times maternal values.

In view of a demonstrated increase in urinary excretion of vitamin B_{12} during pregnancy, the RDA includes the addition of 1 μg/day during pregnancy above the basal requirement of 3 μg/day.

PANTOTHENIC ACID

Pantothenic acid is a portion of coenzyme A, an integral link in the acetylation processes of intermediary metabolism. It is widely distributed in nature, and dietary deficiency has not been demonstrated.

A study in pregnant teenage women found a daily intake of 4.7 mg. This is lower than the average American daily ingestion of 5–20 mg. Blood and urinary excretion levels were also found to be lower in the pregnant teenagers.

Ingestion of 10 mg daily is suggested for pregnant and lactating women. Supplementation with 5–10 mg daily during pregnancy may be required to meet these needs.

ASCORBIC ACID (VITAMIN C)

Humans and other primates, when deprived of vitamin C, develop scurvy, a fatal disease characterized by weaking of collagen. Scurvy still occurs in infants fed only cow's milk and in malnourished and alcoholic adults. Although levels in the fetus are two to three times higher than those in the mother, congenital scurvy has occurred in children born to mothers with the disease. Deficiency of vitamin C has been associated with impaired wound healing. This vitamin is involved in the synthesis of epinephrine and the adrenal steroids.

Ascorbic acid levels progressively decline during pregnancy. Increased levels in the fetus appear to be due to "trapping." The placenta allows passive transfer of dehydroascorbic acid and conversion to the impermeable ascorbic acid in the fetus allows higher concentrations to accumulate.

A great deal of controversy has arisen regarding the intake of large doses of vitamin C in order to prevent the common cold. At present, studies are inconclusive as to the effectiveness of this practice. Theoretical risks include the oxidant effect of large amounts of ascorbic acid in the fetus. In view of these considerations, large doses of vitamin C are not recommended during pregnancy. The RDA includes an intake of 60 mg/day in pregnant women and 80 mg/day in lactating women.

Fat-Soluble Vitamins

VITAMIN A

Dietary vitamin A (retinol) is in the form of preformed vitamin A and carotenoids, especially beta-carotene. Carotenoids must be converted to retinol in order to be useful to the body. Retinol is required for mucous membrane maintenance and as an essential link in the conversion of light energy to nervous activity in the visual process.

Serum vitamin A levels fall in early pregnancy with a subsequent rise early in the second trimester. Levels exceed those of the nonpregnant woman at midpregnancy and rise to approximately 150% of those of nonpregnancy. A slight fall is noted prior to the onset of labor.

The placenta seems to be much more permeable to carotene than to retinol. Levels of retinol of mother and fetus are similar.

Lower levels of carotene in the fetus occur with fetal conversion of carotene to retinol, causing "trapping" of the vitamin.

No effects on the fetus from low levels of vitamin A have been reported. Conversely, experimental hypervitaminosis A has been associated with a variety of congenital anomalies. Although these have been principally seen in experimental animals, a recent report has documented ureteral anomalies in a patient whose mother consumed large doses of vitamin A.

The RDA is 1,000 retinol units during pregnancy. This rise of 20% above the requirement for nonpregnant women allows for fetal storage. In view of the higher doses recommended in some popular literature, vitamin A intake in the pregnant woman should be carefully monitored by the physician.

VITAMIN D

The physiological importance of vitamin D resides in its regulatory role in calcium hemostasis. Vitamin D accelerates intestinal absorption of calcium against an electrochemical gradient and is required for proper bone formation. A deficiency results in rickets in children and osteomalacia in adults.

Vitamin D exists in two forms, D_2 (ergocalciferol) and D_3 (cholecalciferol). D_2 is synthetically produced by the ultraviolet irradiation of the plant sterol ergosterol. D_3 is naturally formed in animal tissue by the exposure of 7-dehydrocholesterol to sunlight. Both forms are equally effective in man. Activity requires conversion of these substrates to the 1,25-dihydrocholecalciferol form sequentially in the liver and kidney.

The level of active forms of vitamin D during pregnancy appears to be related to dietary intake. Values in the fetus seem to reflect the mother's levels, but some regulation via facilitated diffusion probably occurs. This mechanism has been suggested because high levels in the mother have been associated with values in the fetus of 68%–90% of those in the mother, while levels in the fetus of 108% of the mother's values have been noted with low levels in the mother.

The importance of proper vitamin D intake during pregnancy has been documented by the finding of hypocalcemia with low 25-hydroxycholecalciferol levels in premature infants born to mothers with little prenatal care and low serum levels.

Excessive levels of vitamin D intake may contribute to the production of severe maternal and neonatal hypercalcemia. This is especially hazardous with concomitant antacid ingestion.

The RDA does not include an increase during pregnancy above the basal requirement of 400 IU (international units) per day. This quantity of vitamin D is present in 1 quart of fortified milk.

VITAMIN E

Vitamin E has not been shown to be essential for humans. Plasma levels of full-term newborns are about one-third those of adults, and lower levels are found in premature infants. Values in the mother rise during pregnancy to 60% above nonpregnant levels. Since the bulk of plasma vitamin E is carried by serum lipoproteins, the relative concentrations of these substances probably account for these differences.

Although various symptoms have developed in laboratory animals deprived of vitamin E, the only condition associated with deficiency in humans is decreased red blood cell survival time in infants with low birth weight. Studies attempting to raise levels in the fetus to normal adult levels have required 150%–500% over the values of nonpregnant women to achieve this goal. Supplementation has been found to be more effective in the newborn period.

In view of the sparsity of data, the suggested RDA is an intake of 10–20 IU daily since this is present in the diet of an average American. The increase in caloric intake for pregnant and lactating women should account for any additional quantities required by the fetus.

VITAMIN K

The synthesis of coagulation factors II, VII, IX, and X by the liver requires the presence of vitamin K. This vitamin exists in two forms, K_1 (phylloquinone) and K_2 (menaquinone). The former is produced by plants, the latter by bacteria. Menadione, a fat-soluble synthetic product, has approximately twice the biological activity of the natural forms. In view of the production of K_2 by intestinal bacteria, dietary deficiency alone does not exist in the absence of suppression of the flora.

The gut of the newborn contains few bacteria, and the neonate is subject to hemorrhagic tendencies due to relative vitamin K deficiency as well as hepatic immaturity. To a large extent the prolonged prothrombin time seen in the neonate can be normalized by the administration of vitamin K.

In an effort to influence coagulation in the early postnatal period, several investigators have given vitamin K prenatally. The use of large doses of menadione has produced hemolytic anemia in rats and kernicterus in infants of low birth weight. Oral but not intramuscular administration of water-soluble K_1 over the last month of pregnancy has been most effective in improving the neonate's coagulation status.

The current recommendation is 0.5–1 mg of Vitamin K_1 administered intramuscularly to the neonate immediately after birth.

Minerals

IRON

Iron is absorbed primarily in the duodenum and jejunum. Mucosal absorption is affected by gastric juice and gastroferrin, an iron-binding mucoprotein. It is also affected by dietary and pharmacological substances such as phosphates, phylates, and oxalates, which may bind iron in nonabsorable complexes. In the mucosal cell the excess iron absorbed by the intestine is bound as ferritin and shed. This regulatory mechanism usually prevents excess iron accumulation when dietary intake increases.

Approximately 0.5–2.0 mg of iron daily is transported into the bloodstream, where it is bound by transferrin. The transferrin-iron complex circulates, allowing the iron to reach the normoblasts of the bone marrow. In the normoblast, through the action of the enzyme ferrochetolase, an atom of iron is added to protoporphyrin forming heme. The combination of four globin and four heme molecules forms hemoglobin. Iron is also used in the production of myoglobin, cytochromes, and catalases.

Nature has provided an efficient method of conserving iron in the absence of blood loss. Despite an average red blood cell (RBC) lifespan of 120 days, loss of iron is prevented by reutilization. The hemoglobin molecule is broken down in the reticuloendothelial system. The iron molecule is then transferred via transferrin back to the normoblasts in the marrow.

A normal 60-kg woman has about 2.1 gm of iron in her body. A nonpregnant woman has a menstrual loss of 0.5–1.5 mg iron/month as well as a daily loss of about 0.6 mg from the gastrointestinal tract and skin. A pregnant women continues to have the same daily loss. In addition, the average fetus at term contains approximately 200–250 mg of iron while the placenta and cord have another 50 mg. The physiological increase in maternal RBC volume requires an additional 500–600 mg of iron. This leads to a requirement of about 750–900 mg of iron over the course of a pregnancy.

An average American diet contains approximately 6 mg of iron/ 1000 Kcal. Of this iron, approximately 10%–20% is absorbed, depending upon body requirements. Although it would seem that the availability of 0.6–1.2 mg of iron/1000 Kcal is sufficient to meet daily requirements, the demands of growth in adolescence and poor nutrition have led to an incidence of iron deficiency of between 10% and 60% in teenage women.

The need for iron supplementation must be carefully evaluated. Patients with certain disease states such as chronic hemolytic anemias, hemoglobinopathies, and thalassemias must be guarded against indiscriminate iron overload. Observations using bone marrow samples stained for iron stores have shown that 30 mg of oral iron taken daily in the second and third trimesters prevent the depletion of stores during pregnancy.

In patients in whom the diagnosis of iron-deficiency anemia is made, most authorities feel that higher doses are justified in order to obtain normal levels of hemoglobin. Since 34 mg of absorbed iron per day results in maximal response, the recommendation is for 180 mg of oral elemental iron supplementation daily in 3 divided doses.

Many oral iron preparations exist. Standard forms include ferrous sulfate (20% elemental iron), ferrous gluconate (12% elemental iron), and ferrous fumerate (33% elemental iron). Generally the quantity of elemental iron absorbed in iron-deficient states from these inorganic preparations is higher than that found in foods.

The most prominent side effects of oral medicinal iron are related to gastrointestinal intolerance. These include nausea, vomiting, diarrhea, and constipation. Melena, unrelated to gastrointestinal hemorrhage, may develop. It has been recommended that these effects may be minimized with a gradual increase of iron dose up to the amount desired.

Parenteral iron is sometimes prescribed when an iron-deficiency anemia is first discovered during the last few weeks of pregnancy or when the patient cannot be relied upon to take oral iron. It is important to realize when administering parenteral iron that the rapidity of response is essentially the same as occurs with the oral preparations. The major advantage of using parenteral iron is that the total estimated dose required can be delivered to the patient within a few days and one can be assured that the patient has actually received the iron.

The use of parenteral forms of iron must be undertaken with great caution. Anaphylactic reactions, sometimes fatal, occur in association with both intramuscular and intravenous use. There is no evidence that such reactions occur less frequently with intramuscular administration. Other adverse effects that have been reported with use of iron dextran (Imferon®) include severe febrile reactions, reactivation of quiescent rheumatoid arthritis, and phlebitis at the intravenous infusion site.

Intramuscular injections of iron dextran may be less preferable than slow intravenous infusion, as the former often causes pain at the site of injection as well as severe skin discoloration. Iron dextran may also be associated with sarcoma formation at the injection sites.

Iron dextran is given in a total dose of 10–40 ml (500–2,000 mg), according to the patient's calculated needs. The total dose may be diluted in a liter of intravenous fluid and administered slowly for the first 15–30 minutes to detect any allergic reactions, and then more rapidly over 2–6 hours. Alternatively, 0.5 ml may be given intravenously over a 1-minute period, with the remainder of the dose administered slowly after 15–20 minutes. In the latter method, the total dose may be given at one time or it may be divided into 5–10 ml increments over several injections.

CALCIUM

The body of the human adult contains 1,100–1,200 gm of calcium, 99% of which is present in bone. Bone calcium is complexed with phosphate as hydroxyapatite. There is a diurnal flux of about 700 mg daily.

The level of ionized serum calcium is controlled by hormonal and nutritional factors and is maintained in a narrow range. At physiological conditions, approximately 7% of calcium is complexed with citrates and phosphates. The remainder is divided approximately evenly between free and protein-bound forms. Only the free ionized form exerts its physiological effects and is hormonally governed.

The major influences on serum calcium and phosphorus concentration are their solubility products, vitamin-D intake and metabolism, and secretion of the hormones parathormone and calcitonin.

Parathormone is released in response to low or falling levels of ionized calcium. It then acts to increase this level by increasing osteoclast activity, decreasing the renal tubular absorption of phosphate, and augmenting the action of vitamin D in facilitating calcium absorption. High serum levels of ionized calcium cause release of calcitonin, and this hormone inhibits release of calcium from bone.

Vitamin D, in its physiological forms, 1-hydroxycholecalciferol and 1,25-dihydroxycholecalciferol, is essential for the active absorption of calcium from the gut as well as the proper synthesis of bone matrix.

During pregnancy there is an obligatory transfer of approximately 30 gm of calcium to the fetus for mineralization of the skeleton. A number of factors permit this loss by combining to increase intestinal absorption.

Human placental lactogen and high levels of estrogen combine to effect an acceleration of bone metabolism and bone formation. The lower level of ionized calcium produced induces elevation of serum parathormone, which results in a balance of bone formation and resorption, and augments intestinal calcium absorption. This enhancement of bone metabolism and increase in absorption provides an excellent source of calcium that becomes available to the fetus.

The placenta actively transports calcium to the fetus. At full term levels of parathormone in the fetus are low and calcitonin levels high, favoring bone formation.

The calcium reserve in the mother's skeleton is quite high in comparison to needs of the fetus. Although adequate fetal mineralization can occur without calcium supplementation, most authorities feel that the 30 gm loss to the fetus should be replaced. This can be accomplished by adding 300–400 mg of calcium to the 800 mg normal daily requirement. This total of 1,200 mg is fulfilled by drinking 1 quart of milk daily. This amount also provides adequate levels of vitamin D and is sufficient for nursing mothers.

For patients intolerant of milk, similar intake may be provided by means of calcium supplements. In view of the controversial association of leg cramps with high serum phosphorus levels, supplements should probably be in the form of nonphosphorus salts: 500 mg calcium gluconate twice a day should suffice.

ZINC

Zinc is essential as a cofactor for many enzyme systems in plants and animals. Although the body contains relatively large amounts of zinc stored in bone, these supplies are not metabolically active. Dietary deficiency leads to loss of appetite and failure to grow. Gross zinc deficiency seen in the Middle East results in hypogonadism and dwarfism. Intrauterine deficiency, even when temporary, has resulted in permanent anomalies in experimental animals.

Marginal zinc deficiency seems to exist in the United States, usually in areas with low soil levels of zinc. Giving supplements to children with marginal deficiency has resulted in increased taste acuity, improved appetite, and greater growth.

Congenital lesions of the central nervous system appear to be greater in geographical areas in which zinc deficiency exists. Recent studies have revealed that zinc is an essential component of the bacterial inhibitory system of the amniotic fluid. There is some suggestion that dietary availability of zinc may alter the effectiveness of this system.

Total body zinc increases throughout pregnancy. Levels at full term are approximately 50% above those of nonpregnant women. Plasma and hair concentrations, however, fall during this period.

The zinc content of the diet of an average adult American is 10–25 mg. Metabolic studies have revealed that balance can be maintained with an intake of 8–10 mg daily in the nonpregnant state.

Despite the important implications of the above-mentioned observations, little data are available on the maintenance of homeostasis in the pregnant woman. The RDA includes an additional 15 mg/day during pregnancy, above basal recommendations of 15 mg/day. This may indicate a need for supplementation. Of the commonly prescribed vitamin preparations, 15 mg per capsule is contained in Natalins Rx® and One-A-Day Plus Minerals®.

CHROMIUM

Interest in chromium metabolism in pregnancy has centered around its role in glucose utilization. Chromium deficiency can be associated with decreased glucose tolerance, and its supplementation has ameliorated glucose intolerance in some clinical states. Studies have revealed lower serum concentrations during pregnancy than in the nonpregnant state. Gravid patients have failed to respond to a glucose load with the decrease in chromium level noted in nonpregnant subjects. The relationship of these findings to the impaired glucose utilization characteristic of pregnancy is unknown at this time.

IODINE

Iodine is required in the formation of the thyroid hormones, throxine and triiodothyronine. Iodine deficiency leads to goiter formation. For nonpregnant adult women the minimal requirement necessary to prevent goiter formation is approximately 1 μg/kg of body weight. The RDA for iodine is between 100 and 300 μg/day.

The most efficient method of obtaining this amount is through iodized salt, which contains 76 μg of iodine per gram. Since iodized salt is rarely used in commercially prepared foods, it is recommended that this preparation be used as added table salt.

It should be noted that pharmacological doses of iodides may cause goiter formation in the fetus.

COPPER

Copper is essential for all mammals. In rare instances copper dietary deficiency has occurred in humans, leading to anemia, neutropenia, and bone disease. In experimental animals with copper deficiencies, major anomalies have been produced due to defective cross-linking in elastin and collagen. The fetus requires copper, and it accumulates in certain fetal organs in much greater concentrations than are seen in adult tissue. The copper concentration in the fetal liver, for example, is 5 to 10 times that of an adult.

Copper intake of 2 mg/day seems to maintain a homeostatic balance in adults. Serum levels in the fetus rise throughout pregnancy. This may be related to elevated levels of estrogen since the increase of the two is coincident. Furthermore, exogenous estrogens raise serum levels of copper in nonpregnant women.

Multivitamin Preparations

Table 14 is a list of those multivitamin preparations most commonly dispensed from the Yale–New Haven Medical Center Pharmacy. As mentioned in the text, supplementation of zinc and pantothenic acid may be required during pregnancy. Of the commonly used prenatal preparations containing 30 mg of iron or more, only Natalins Rx contains zinc.

Table 14. Vitamin and Mineral Content of Selected Multivitamin Preparations

Preparation	Iron	Folate	Vitamin B_6	Vitamin D	Calcium	Pantothenic Acid	Zinc
One-A-Day®	0	0.4 mg	2.0 mg	400 IU	0	0	0
One-A-Day + Iron®	18 mg	0.4 mg	2.0 mg	400 IU	0	0	0
One-A-Day + Minerals®	18 mg	0.4 mg	2.0 mg	400 IU	100 mg	10 mg	15 mg
Theragran®	0	0	3.3 mg	400 IU	0	20 mg	0
Natalins®	45 mg	0.8 mg	4.0 mg	400 IU	200 mg	0	0
Natalins Rx®	60 mg	1.0 mg	10 mg	400 IU	200 mg	15 mg	15 mg
Stuart Prenatal®	60 mg	0.8 mg	4.0 mg	400 IU	200 mg	0	0
Stuartnatal®	65 mg	1.0 mg	10 mg	400 IU	200 mg	0	0

RECOMMENDED READING

Bernhardt, I. B., and Dorsey, D. J.   Hypervitaminosis A and congenital renal anomalies in a human fetus. *Obstet. Gynecol.* 43:750–755, 1974.

Brzezinski, A., Bromberg, Y. M., and Braun, K.   Riboflavin excretion during pregnancy and early lactation. *J. Lab. Clin. Med.* 39:84–90, 1952.

Cleary, R. E., Lumeng, L., and Li, T.   Maternal and fetal plasma levels of pyridoxal phosphate at term: Adequacy of vitamin B_6 supplementation during pregnancy. *Am. J. Obstet. Gynecol.* 121:25–28, 1975.

Coursin, D. B., and Brown, V. C.   Changes in vitamin B_6 during pregnancy. *Am. J. Obstet. Gynecol.* 82:1307–1311, 1961.

Davidson, I. W., and Burt, R. L.   Physiologic changes in plasma chromium of normal and pregnant women: Effect of a glucose load. *Am. J. Obstet. Gynecol.* 116:601–608, 1973.

Dokumov, S. I.   Serum copper and pregnancy. *Am. J. Obstet. Gynecol.* 101:217–222, 1968.

Greenberg, G.   Sarcoma after intramuscular iron injection. *Br. Med. J.* 1:1508–1509, 1976.

Heller, S., Salkeld, R. M., and Korner, W. F.   Riboflavin status in pregnancy. *Am. J. Clin. Nutr.* 27:1225–1230, 1974.

Heller, S., Salkeld, R. M., and Korner, W. F.   Vitamin B_1 status in pregnancy. *Am. J. Clin. Nutr.* 27:1221–1224, 1974.

Kitay, D. Z., and Harbort, M. S.   Iron and folic acid deficiency in pregnancy. *Clin. Perinatol.* 2:255–273, 1975.

Lundin, P. M.   The carcinogenic action of complex iron preparations. *Br. J. Cancer* 15:838–847, 1961.

Malone, J. M.   Vitamin passage across the placenta. *Clin. Perinatol.* 2:295–307, 1975.

Owen, G. M., Nelson, C. E., Baker, G. L., Connor, W. E., and Jacobs, J. P.   Use of vitamin K_1 in pregnancy. *Am. J. Obstet. Gynecol.* 99:368–373, 1967.

Pitkin, R. M.   Calcium metabolism in pregnancy: A review. *Am. J. Obstet. Gynecol.* 121:724–737, 1975.

Pitkin, R. M.   Vitamins and minerals in pregnancy. *Clin. Perinatol.* 2:221–232, 1975.

Recommended Daily Allowances   (8th ed.). Washington, D.C.: National Academy of Science, 1974.

Schlievert, P., Johnson, W., and Galask, R. P.   Bacterial growth inhibition by the amnionic fluid: VII. The effect of zinc supplementation on bacterial inhibitory activity of amnionic fluids from gestation of 20 weeks. *Am. J. Obstet. Gynecol.* 127:603–608, 1977.

Scott, D. E., and Pritchard, J. A.   Anemia in pregnancy. *Clin. Perinatol.* 1:491–506, 1974.

(WOB)

Drug Classification Index

Generic and Trade Name Index